Nursing Leadership and Management: A Practical Guide

Patricia L. Carroll RN, BC, CEN, RRT, MS
Educational Medical Consultants
Meriden, CT

Health Careers Program
Maloney High School
Meridien, CT

THOMSON
⎯⎯✳⎯⎯ ™
DELMAR LEARNING   Australia · Canada · Mexico · Singapore · Spain · United Kingdom · United States

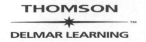

THOMSON
DELMAR LEARNING

Nursing Leadership and Management: A Practical Guide
by Patricia L. Carroll

Vice President,
Health Care Business Unit:
William Brottmiller

Director of Learning Solutions:
Matthew Kane

Acquisitions Editor:
Tamara Caruso

Editorial Assistant:
Tiffiny Adams

Marketing Director:
Jennifer McAvey

Marketing Channel Manager:
Michele McTighe

Marketing Coordinator:
Danielle Pacella

Production Director:
Carolyn Miller

Production Manager:
Barbara A. Bullock

Production Editor:
Jack Pendleton

Library of Congress Cataloging-in-Publication Data

Carroll, Patricia, 1958-
   Nursing leadership and management : a practical guide / Patricia L. Carroll.
      p. ; cm.
   Includes bibliographical references.
   ISBN 1-4018-2704-7
   1. Nursing services— Administration.
   2. Leadership.
   [DNLM: 1. Leadership— Handbooks. 2. Nursing, Supervisory— Handbooks.
   3. Nurse's Role— Handbooks.
   4. Nursing Care— organization & administration— Handbooks.
   5. Personnel Management— Handbooks. WY 49 C319n 2005] I. Title.
      RT89.C32 2005
      362.17'3068—dc22
                        200502672

This book is dedicated to all my students past, present, and future...from whom I have learned so much.

CONTENTS

Preface   vii

About the Author   ix

Reviewer List   x

Part I: INTRODUCTION TO NURSING LEADERSHIP   **1**

1   What is Leadership?   2

2   What is Management?   18

3   Leadership Versus Management   30

4   A Positive Definition of Power   40

5   Accountability in Nursing Leadership   53

Part II: PRIMARY SKILLS FOR THE NURSING LEADER   **61**

6   What is Communication?   62

7   Communication Skills   80

8   Decision-Making and Time-Management Tools   92

9   Change Management Skills   109

10   Conflict Resolution Skills   125

11   Team Building Skills   138

Part III: PUTTING THE PRIMARY SKILLS TO WORK: STRATEGIC ORGANIZATIONAL ROLES FOR THE NURSING LEADER   **151**

12   Managing First-Line Patient Care   152

13   Strategic Thinking to Improve Patient Care (Including Evidence-Based Care)   163

14 Managing Patient Care and Outcomes Through
Improving Organization Quality   174

15 Managing and Supporting Excellence in Staff Performance   186

16 Nurses as Professional Leaders Inside and Outside
the Health Care Organization   201

Part IV: THE HEALTH CARE ENVIRONMENT AND ITS IMPACT ON NURSING LEADERSHIP   211

17 Current Health Care Environment (and into the Future)   212

18 Nursing Leaders Influencing Politics and Acting
as Patient Advocates   231

19 Nursing Leadership and Collective Bargaining   241

20 Delegation   253

21 Current and Future Opportunities for Nurse Leaders   267

Part V: LEGAL AND ETHICAL ASPECTS OF NURSING LEADERSHIP   277

22 Legal Aspects of Nursing Leadership   278

23 Ethical Issues in Nursing Leadership   296

Part VI: PUTTING IT ALL TOGETHER AND BECOMING A NURSING LEADER   305

24 Ten Ways to Become a Leader   306

Answer Key   310
Index   314

PREFACE

"Leadership and learning are indispensable to each other"

This phrase comes from the speech John F. Kennedy was going to deliver in Dallas the day he was assassinated. The speech stressed that, "leadership must be guided by the lights of learning and reason..." Kennedy's focus was on America's leadership in the world, but the same principles apply to America's nursing leaders. You cannot be a nursing leader without a commitment to lifelong learning.

I have written this book because I feel passionately about nursing leadership. It's critically important to understand that leadership is a personal choice – it is not bestowed on someone with a job title. Being in a position of authority does not automatically make you a leader. There are nurse managers who are not leaders, just as there are staff nurses who are powerful leaders.

Leadership is a process of influence. Leaders can have a positive impact simply by personal example. A leader can be a staff nurse who reaches out to and supports new grads when other staff members reject less experienced nurses. A nurse can be a leader by publishing a case study about an unusual patient situation in order to educate others. And a nurse who volunteers at a homeless shelter can be a leader in patient advocacy.

Nurse leaders should consider their role within the larger context of the nursing profession and how nursing is presented to the public. When my first book for consumers, "What Nurses Know and Doctors Don't Have Time to Tell You," was published in 2004, I did a lot of interviews—for magazines, newspapers, radio and television. Inevitably, the first question was, "So what is it that nurses know?" And my answer was, "Nurses focus their practice on treating *how people respond* to illness, injuries and a variety of conditions. Physicians, on the other hand, are taught to focus on the diseases themselves." I was able to be an advocate for the nursing profession; to teach readers, listeners, and viewers about the difference between nursing and medical practice; and to empower them by sharing information about their health.

I am now a columnist for the New York Daily News. My column, "What Nurses Know" appears on Wednesdays, and I get terrific questions from readers. Many write about how glad they are to be able to contact a nurse. When I write, I think about helping readers to become educated and informed so they can make their own decisions. I think of it as the ultimate patient teaching opportunity— to teach 750,000 New Yorkers each week. As I write each column, I am mindful that I have the platform from which I can positively influence readers' opinions of nurses.

Thus, this book focuses on the qualities of leadership, roles of influence, and the responsibilities of nurse leaders.

Nursing Leadership and Management: A Practical Guide is designed to be used two ways: as a text for traditional nursing programs that prefer using a hand-book on leadership rather than a full textbook, or as a comprehensive overview of leadership for nurses in nontraditional nursing degree programs and those reviewing for a class or the NCLEX exam.

Each part of each section follows the same format to enhance learning:

- Key terms (which are highlighted when first used in the text)
- Content in outline form, focusing on practical, need-to-know information
- Multiple choice review questions in NCLEX format
- Thinking questions that encourage you to apply key concepts
- Discussion questions for classroom assignments or study group work
- Print reference list and suggested readings
- Webliography to encourage you to explore the latest trends and issues online
- Answers to multiple choice questions in the back of the book so you can check your work

I have never been a department manager, nor have I been elected to office in a nursing organization. However, because I have spent the past 20 years trav-eling all over the country teaching at conferences and conventions, caring for patients, writing articles to teach others, and proudly representing my profes-sion in the national media, I have been called a nursing leader. There is no other professional title I carry more proudly. Now I have started a new chapter in my professional life by leading the health careers program at my local high school. It is an incredible opportunity to prepare the health care leaders of the future.

I'd like to hear from you and learn what you liked best about this book, what you'd like to see added, or what you've had trouble with. You can visit my Web site at http://www.nursesnotebook.com or e-mail me at pat@nursesnotebook. com.

Here's to your success!

Patricia Carroll, RN, BC, CEN, RRT, MS
Meriden, CT Winter, 2006

ABOUT THE AUTHOR

Patricia Carroll has more than 20 years experience in health care, as both a registered respiratory therapist and a registered nurse. She has worked in neonatal, pediatric, and adult critical care; emergency nursing; high-tech home care; and community health. She is board certified in emergency nursing, general nursing practice, and nursing professional development. Pat is an award-winning medical writer; this is her fourth book.

Pat is currently the Health Careers program coordinator at Maloney High School in Meriden, CT.

REVIEWER LIST

Deborah Brabham, RN, BSN
Florida Community College Jacksonville
Jacksonville, FL

Daryl Boucher, MS, RN
Northern Maine Community College
Presque Isle, ME

Pam Cook, RN, MSN, CNA, COI
Medical College of Georgia
Augusta, GA

Diane Faucher Moy, MSN, RN, APRN-BC, CNS
University of Texas at Austin
Austin, TX

Becky Haglund, RN, MN
Santa Ana College
Irvine, CA

Diane Johnson, RN, BSN, MS, DNC
Chattanooga State Technical Community College
Chattanooga, TN

Patricia Newland, RN, BS, MS
Broome Community College
Binghamton, NY

Part I
Introduction to Nursing Leadership

CHAPTER

1

WHAT IS LEADERSHIP?

KEY TERMS

authority
autocratic leadership
charismatic theory
contingency theories
curiosity
democratic leadership
desire
employee-centered leadership
empowerment
flexibility
formal leadership
informal leadership
integrity
intelligence

laissez-faire leadership
leader
leadership
leadership theories
motivational theories
new leadership concept
passion
positive interaction
process of influence
reciprocal
self-confidence
support
transformational leadership theory
vision

INTRODUCTION

Leadership, defined as a process of influence, is not limited to people who occupy traditional positions of authority. Any person in an organization can be a leader. However, all leaders tend to possess a number of similar characteristics, including passion, integrity, curiosity, flexibility, intelligence, ability to support others, and self-confidence. A number of theories have been developed over time that attempt to explain different leadership types and evaluate their effectiveness. Current theories focus on leader behaviors that allow organizations to respond to rapidly changing environments—particularly relevant to the field of health care.

KEY POINTS

1. Leadership: definition

   A.   **Leadership** is defined as a **process of influence.**

   B.   Leadership is not limited to people in traditional positions of authority. Similarly, leadership is not automatic when a nurse is in an authoritative position.

   C.   A **leader** influences others to move in the direction of achieving goals.

   D.   Leadership can occur in a number of dynamics and settings.

       i.   A leader can influence one person.

      ii.   A leader can influence more than one person, including small and large groups, organizations, even entire communities or societies.

2. For leadership to be successful, the following characteristics must be present.

   A.   There must be **positive interactions** between leaders and followers.

   B.   The leaders and followers must have a **reciprocal** relationship (communication, ideas, and respect—must move back and forth, not just from the top-down).

3. True leadership is not based on "traditional" views of leadership as having authority, command, or power over others.

   A.   Leaders can take charge of a situation, but taking charge and being responsible are not the only characteristics of leadership.

   B.   Leadership and a position of **authority** are not equivalent.

       i.   A person in a position of authority is not automatically a leader.

      ii.   Ideally, nurses in positions of authority have highly developed leadership qualities.

4. Types of leadership

   A.   **Formal** leader: A formal leader is a person in a position of influence or authority or who has a sanctioned role within an organization.

   B.   **Informal** leader: An informal leader is a person who demonstrates leadership and has influence even though he or she is not in a formal leadership role in an organization.
Informal leadership is marked by two key traits:

       i.   Ability to influence others.

      ii.   Other people in the group or organization recognize that ability and are influenced.

5. Core traits of leaders: Research on leadership does not reveal any absolute qualities that define a leader, but most experts agree that effective leaders have the following core values (see Bennis and Nanus, 1985; McCall, 1998):

    A.   A guiding **vision**

        i. A leader is able to *see* a picture of the desired future.

        ii. Such a picture allows the leader to set goals toward that desired future.

    B.   **Passion**

        i. A leader is enthusiastic about the future possibilities.

        ii. He or she has the ability to inspire people and align them in a common effort to make those future possibilities a reality.

    C.   **Integrity**

        i. Leaders who have integrity possess a significant knowledge of the self or self-awareness, including knowledge of their strengths and weaknesses and the ability to receive feedback and learn from mistakes.

        ii. Integrity requires honesty and maturity.

        iii. It is supported by the inner strength of the person's convictions and his or her ability to deal with conflict or obstacles that arise.

        iv. A leader's integrity is developed through personal and professional experience and growth.

        v. Having integrity means that the person can be trusted.

    D.   **Curiosity** and/or daring

        i. Leaders draw on these traits to enable them to take risks.

        ii. These traits facilitate change.

        iii. These traits also shorten the learning curve because leaders intuitively zero in on *what works* rather than wasting time on *what doesn't work*.

6. Additional traits commonly found in leaders: In addition to the core traits discussed earlier, numerous researchers have found the following traits commonly attributed to leaders.

    A.   **Flexibility**

        i. This trait allows leaders to adapt rapidly to changes in all aspects of the environment. In nursing, this can mean being able to manage six new admissions on the same shift (small scale) to merging nursing units as part of a hospital-wide redesign (large scale).

      ii. Flexibility also allows leaders to deal effectively and creatively with uncertainty and even hostility that may come their way.

B. **Intelligence**

      i. *Subject-based intelligence* includes knowledge and skills associated with the person's job functions, and the ability to use the knowledge and skills to solve problems and improve work processes.

      ii. *People-based intelligence* includes "emotional intelligence"—the ability to use not only rational but also emotional perception in learning, problem-solving, and working with people effectively to achieve desired outcomes. Note that in nursing, this not only yields positive patient outcomes, but also results in the ongoing professional development and job satisfaction of the nurse.

C. Ability to **support** others. This trait includes the following characteristics:

      i. Responsiveness to a wide range of situations and people. A person with this trait is likely to face situations head-on rather than withdrawing or procrastinating.

      ii. The leader who is able to support others practices open and effective communication.

      iii. The leader who is able to support others possesses key social skills—the ability to work effectively with and respect diverse constituents, to defuse conflict, and to generate trust and enthusiasm in others.

D. **Self-confidence**

      i. A person who is self-confident is able to trust his or her abilities and decisions.

      ii. This person is also able to receive feedback and input from others without feeling threatened.

E. **Desire** to lead. According to Kirkpatrick and Locke (1991), people who are effective leaders must be interested in and have a desire to influence change in people or organizations.

F. Does gender matter?

      i. Leadership and management characteristics, styles, and behaviors have historically been seen as "masculine" because most people in management were men. Current research draws a variety of conclusions about the impact of gender on nursing:

        a. gender differences do occur and impact the workplace (Rudan, 2003; Davidhizar & Cramer, 2000)

        b. these differences, however, can be used to provide balanced and multifaceted teams (Rudan, 2003)

      c. interestingly, a study of female and male nurse executives showed that most favored gender-neutral leadership characteristics over those characterized as traditionally masculine or feminine (Rozier, 1996)

    ii. How people perceive gender traits in the workplace is strongly impacted by which gender is in the majority. Male and female business leaders tend to adopt characteristics of the dominant male leadership while male and female nurses tend to adopt characteristics of the dominant female leadership (Rozier, 1996).

7. **Leadership theories**. Through the years, a number of researchers have developed theories about leadership, which are discussed next. Be aware that older theories were developed based on the study of white men. These may or may not apply to women and people of color.

   A.   Behavioral theories. These theories were developed by Kurt Lewin and his colleagues at Iowa State University, beginning in the 1930s. Many are still recognized and accepted even today.

       i. **Autocratic leadership**: This type of leadership is based on centralized decision making. The leader makes decisions and expects subordinates to obey. This leader uses his or her power to command others and to control them. This type of leadership may produce significant results, such as in the military, but generally is not seen as a long-term effective leadership style. If this type of leadership style is used consistently, a great deal of hostility may develop between the leader and the followers.

      ii. **Laissez-faire leadership**: With this leadership style, the leader defers decision making to her or his followers. The opposite of the autocratic leader, the laissez-faire leader is often permissive and tends to be distant or uninvolved. Workers in this situation may wind up feeling frustrated (because the person who is supposed to make decisions does not), and efficiency may suffer as a result.

     iii. **Democratic leadership**: In this type of leadership, the leader allows others to participate in decision making and to share authority. The leader's power is derived from his or her expertise as well as the leverage that results from close relationships with others. This type of group tends to perform well whether or not the leader is present, and leaders and followers tend to maintain positive relationships.

     iv. **Employee-centered leadership**: With this leadership style, the focus is on the human needs of the employees. Employee-centered leadership is considered more effective than job-focused leadership, which is more concerned with schedules, tasks, or output than with the people who do the work.

B. **Contingency theories**. The *contingency approaches to leadership* state
    that a variety of environmental factors affect the outcome as much as
    do leadership style or leader characteristics. In other words, the out-
    comes of leadership are determined by factors other than the leader's
    behavior. These contingency theories are discussed below.

    i. Fielder's theory. According to this theory, leader behavior
        depends on the interaction of the leader's personality and the
        particular needs of the situation. According to this theory (see
        Fielder, 1967), leadership effectiveness depends on matching
        organizational structure with the best leadership style for that
        organization and situation. According to Fielder, leadership
        effectiveness consists of the three following characteristics:
        a. Leader-member relations: These include the followers' feel-
            ings about the leader, including the level of trust, acceptance
            of the leader, and whether the leader is perceived as credible
            by his or her followers.
        b. Task structure: This includes the extent to which work tasks
            are defined by specific procedures, directions, and goals. Tasks
            are classified as high structure (routine, clearly defined) or low
            structure (not predictable, creative, working "on the fly"). This
            concept could also be applied to a work environment. For
            example, postpartum is generally predictable with stable
            patients compared to the emergency department's complete
            lack of routine.
        c. Position power: This includes the amount of influence and/or
            the degree of formal authority that the leader has. In this
            model, high position power is considered favorable while low
            position power is considered less so.
    ii. Hersey and Blanchard's situational theory. According to this
         theory, the effectiveness of a person's leadership style depends
         not so much on the leader but on the follower—the follower's
         maturity should be assessed in order for the most appropriate
         leadership style to be implemented. With this leadership style,
         the effective leader also changes or adapts her or his leader-
         ship style to match the followers' needs and attempts to increase
         the followers' level of maturity. This leadership style can be
         categorized in four ways (based on task and relationship
         levels):
         a. high task/low relationship behavior: "telling" leadership style
         b. high task/high relationship behavior: "selling" leadership
             style (getting people to "buy in" to an approach, policy, or
             new staffing or management structure)
         c. low task/high relationship behavior: "participating" leadership
             style

> d. low task/low relationship behavior: "delegating" leadership style

iii. House's path-goal theory: According to this theory, the effective leader makes the appropriate path easier for the worker to follow by using the appropriate leadership style. The effective leader also matches his or her leadership style to the situation or environment, for example, the type or complexity of tasks that need to be completed and the dynamics of work groups. According to this theory, when the leader aligns leadership style with followers' needs and the particular situation, he or she enhances worker performance and satisfaction. As Northouse (2001) points out, the path-goal theory has its roots in expectancy theory, which says that people are motivated by being able to carry out their work, which they believe will contribute to the desired outcome and provide them with rewards for that work.

In nursing, for example, a manager might need very different approaches: in a long-term care facility in which there is a predominance of non-RN staff, with many certified nurses' aides, a manager may need to be more hands-on and delegate fewer tasks and responsibilities. On the other hand, an all-RN staff in a high-technology, high acuity critical care setting may be able to function more independently, meaning the manager can delegate more and the staff can be active participants in management decisions. A mismatch in which independent nurses are given a hands-on manager, or a situation in which less skilled workers do not get enough direct supervision can lead to significant frustration among all nursing staff members and may affect the quality of patient care delivered.

iv. Kerr and Jermier's "substitutes for leadership" theory: According to this theory, certain variables or factors may influence followers' behaviors as much as or even more than the leader's behavior. Some of these identified substitutes for leader behavior include:

> a. amount of feedback provided by the task itself (for example, the difference between taking care of a patient in a coma versus a patient who communicates and actively participates in care)
>
> b. significant work group cohesion (do experienced nurses make it difficult for less experienced nurses to be part of "the group"?)
>
> c. group's rigid adherence to rules (not only formal, but informal rules as well, such as whether nurses are expected to take personal responsibility for continuing education or if professional development is not valued)
>
> d. intrinsic satisfaction provided by the work or task

For example, when critical care nurses are rotated out of critical care to a high-tech chronic care unit, nurses' job satisfaction may drop because the nurses experience much less feedback from their work;

patients' conditions do not change rapidly in response to nursing interventions as they do in critical care. Rotation out of the original work environment can dilute group cohesion, and the nurses may not feel intrinsic satisfaction from this type of work compared to their usual fast-paced critical care work.

C. Current contemporary theories. The most contemporary leadership theories address leader behaviors or functions that are needed to develop "learning organizations" and allow organizations to change or transform themselves according to the changes in their environment. The two major contemporary theories of leadership are the charismatic and transformational theories.

  i. **Charismatic theory**: According to House (1977), leaders who have charisma (leadership qualities that inspire followers' allegiance and devotion) are able to make an emotional connection with their followers. Generally, these leaders display enormous self-confidence and are able to get others to have confidence in them. The positive aspect of the charismatic leader is his or her ability to communicate vision and use unconventional strategies effectively (especially in a crisis). President John F. Kennedy used this type of leadership by showing his self-confidence in an unconventional strategy for the time—by appearing on television. This was especially important during the Cuban missile crisis when the United States faced the threat of nuclear war after the Soviet Union placed nuclear missiles in Cuba. On the other hand, some followers may assign a sort of "superhuman" quality or purpose to the charismatic leader, which has allowed some charismatic leaders such as Adolph Hitler and Charles Manson to do great harm.

  ii. **Transformational leadership theory**: With this type of leadership, both leaders and followers act on one another to raise their motivation and performance to higher levels. This theory depends on the concept of **empowerment**, in which all parties are allowed to work together, to the best of their ability, to achieve a collective goal. This process transforms both the leader and the follower. The focus of transformational leadership is allowing innovation and change. According to this theory, there are two types of leaders:

  a. transactional leader: the person responsible for day-to-day operations.

  b. transformational leader: the person responsible for maintaining the overall vision and motivating people to incorporate that vision in their work.

D. **Motivational theories**: These theories are sometimes called *process* theories because they are designed to do more than just explain behavior.

They are designed to help us understand the processes involved in people's behavior. The four key motivational theories are discribed below.

i. Reinforcement theory: This theory, based on the research of B.F. Skinner (1953), views motivation as learning. Through this process, a person becomes conditioned to associate a behavior with a consequence (either a positive or a negative reinforcement). According to this theory, leaders are most effective when they can control or even manipulate the consequences of a follower's behavior. This behavior-modification approach works well when enough positive reinforcements exist and when leaders have a certain control over followers' access to these rewards.

This theory does not explain, however, why some reinforcements work for some people and not for others. In some cases, rewards can divide staff if the same people tend to get rewards over and over again, and some nurses are insulted by the concept of rewards, such as a free lunch coupon or other small tokens. The efficacy of this approach may also be affected by a person's educational background, age, and cultural experiences.

ii. Expectancy theory: This theory moves a step beyond Skinner's behavior modification approach, noting that people's expectations about a situation also help determine their behavior. Expectancy theory emphasizes that people don't just respond passively to reinforcement or lack thereof; rather, they are actively and consciously interacting with their environment. Proponents of this theory often construct a matrix that helps quantify the following three motivational components:
   a. expectancy: the perceived probability that a certain effort will lead to a desired action or behavior.
   b. instrumentality: the belief that a given performance level will lead to an outcome.
   c. valence: perceived value of that outcome.

In nursing, the "expectation" is often one of being taken for granted, being overworked and not receiving recognition for extra effort or a job well done. Thus, nurses may decide not to "go the extra mile" if they expect that their efforts will not be acknowledged or appreciated. A true nursing leader can change these expectations by keeping the focus on the patient and family outcomes and the self-satisfaction that comes from prioritizing their needs. A nursing leader can help staff nurses develop the ability to achieve satisfaction from the intrinsic rewards of their work, altering their expectations for external rewards.

iii. Equity theory: This theory says that the degree of perceived fairness in the work situation is the key to job satisfaction and worker effort. Note that equity does not mean equality—it is still possible, for example, for workers with different skill levels, different levels of educational preparation, or different levels of seniority in the workplace to receive different pay. What is important is that the workers perceive that they are receiving a fair and just reward for their efforts, and that their efforts are being rewarded proportionately to the efforts of other workers. Workers who perceive that inequity exists will usually modify their work (usually in terms of amount of work or difficulty of work) in order to restore equity themselves.

    iv. Goal setting theory: This theory, in contrast to expectancy and equity theories, suggests that people don't expend effort for rewards or task outcomes, but to accomplish the goal itself. According to Locke (1968), three assumptions form the foundation of this theory:

        a. specific goals are more effective than general goals for motivating higher performance

        b. more difficult or challenging goals lead to higher performance

        c. incentives or rewards are effective only in that they encourage people to change their goals (that is, it's not the reward in itself that promotes improvement)

E.   Wheatley's "**new leadership**" concept: According to this theory developed by Margaret Wheatley (1992), the leader's function in an organization is to:

    i. use his or her vision to guide followers

    ii. help followers make choices based on values shared by leaders and followers

    iii. provide meaning and coherence in the organizational culture

This leadership concept draws strongly on the biological concept of organisms, contending that, like an organism, the organization is a living entity whose different parts are interdependent on each other for the entire organization to thrive. This theory sees the organization as being able to form strong internal connections and balances that promote the best functioning — an environment that provides optimal patient outcomes through collaboration in the workplace and maximizes worker satisfaction.

F.   Gender studies have noted that the qualities of a so-called feminine approach to leadership (more than 95% of nurses are female) have the following characteristics:

    i. flexible interconnections are valued more than rigid hierarchies

    ii. power and information are seen as a shared, nonfinite commodity

    iii. emphasis is less on competition or "winning" than on relation, participation, facilitating, nurturing, and diversity

G. How do changes in organizations engender changes in leadership theory and practice?

    i. Organizations today are more complex, and leadership styles and methods must keep pace with the complexities of people, the patient care they provide, and the technology they use.

    ii. The most effective leadership emerges from teams that are able to direct and organize themselves.

    iii. Leaders must be able to lead teams that are diverse in terms of gender, race, culture, and age and deal effectively with the different needs and motivations of these groups.

REVIEW ACTIVITIES

Questions

1. Leadership is best defined as a process of

a. coercion
b. interpersonal dynamics
c. influence
d. passive learning

2. A person who is a leader but who does not have a sanctioned role within the organization is what kind of leader?

a. formal
b. informal
c. situational
d. traditional

3. The leadership trait defined as self-knowledge or self-awareness and the ability to receive feedback and learn from mistakes is called

a. passion
b. vision
c. curiosity
d. integrity

4. The trait that allows leaders to adapt rapidly to changes in the organization's environment is called

a. support
b. intelligence
c. self-confidence
d. flexibility

5. A leader who defers decision making to his or her followers is called what type of leader?

    a.   autocratic
    b.   laissez-faire
    c.   contingency
    d.   high task

6. Which group of leadership theories states that the leader's style has less impact on outcomes than on certain environmental and other factors?

    a.   contingency theory
    b.   democracy theory
    c.   charismatic theory
    d.   goal-setting theory

7. According to House's path-goal theory, which of the following is true?

    a.   effectiveness of leadership style depends more on the follower than the leader
    b.   the leader's effective leadership style helps the worker remain on the appropriate path
    c.   the leader's charisma or personal appeal helps workers remain on the appropriate path
    d.   workers are empowered to achieve a common purpose

8. The theory that maintains that followers and leaders influence each other to increase their motivation and performance to higher levels is called

    a.   reinforcement theory
    b.   equity theory
    c.   goal-setting theory
    d.   transformational leadership theory

9. The concept of valence is defined as

    a.   the perceived probability that a certain effort will lead to a desired action or behavior
    b.   the belief that a certain effort will lead to a desired action
    c.   perceived value of an outcome
    d.   behavior that is repeated because it is positively or negatively reinforced

10. The "new leadership" theory was proposed by

    a.   Skinner
    b.   Wheatley
    c.   Locke
    d.   Bennis

Critical-Thinking Questions

1. A sudden ice storm struck at about 9:30 on a Thursday night. There were multiple motor vehicle crashes, and the community hospital emergency department was overwhelmed with injured patients. At the same time, two people having massive heart attacks arrived by ambulance for care. The evening shift staff was scheduled to go home at 11:30 p.m. All staff, except for two people, stayed to help the night shift, not leaving until 3:00 a.m. The two people who left angered the rest of the staff because they did not pitch in to help, and offered no explanation for leaving. The following day, the evening staff arrived to see a memo posted in the staff lounge from the nurse manager thanking the staff for staying late, pitching in, and "going the extra mile" for the patients, their coworkers, and the department. However, the memo was addressed to the people who were on the staffing list for the evening shift, and included the two people who left early. Using one or more of the theories described in this chapter, describe the positive and negative aspects of the nurse manager's behavior.

2. An enthusiastic, 28-year-old nurse is promoted to the nurse manager's position on a different nursing unit within the same hospital. She worked on an oncology unit, and is now manager of a mixed medical-surgical unit that uses critical paths extensively for its orthopedic surgical patients. She is the third new manager in 3 years.

   Every nurse who works on the day shift in this unit has been there for 10 years or more. When the new manager spent some time on the unit observing the activities before taking the job, Mary, a nurse with 15 years of service to the hospital, stood out from the rest of the staff members. She told people what to do, and decided who went to break and lunch at what times. She called staff members together for report at the end of the shift.

   What challenges does this "new" nurse manager face?

Discussion Questions

1. What leadership style or styles do you observe in the leaders you interact with?
2. What leadership style do you think you are more inclined to use? Does your style change in different situations? Why or why not?
3. Do you think that one leadership style is better than the other(s)? Why or why not?
4. Analyze the leadership style of the director of your nursing school. What theories apply? What positive and negative aspects have you experienced from your director's leadership style?

5. Make a list of three nursing leaders you know personally, have met, or know about. What makes these people "leaders?"

Works Cited

Bennis, W., & Nanus, B. (1985). *Leaders: The strategies for taking charge.* New York: Harper & Row.

Costello-Nickitas, D. (1997). *Quick reference to nursing leadership.* Albany, NY: Thomson Delmar Learning.

Davidhizar, R. & Cramer, C. (2000). Gender differences in leadership in the health professions. *Health Care Manager, 18*(3), 18–24.

Fielder, F. (1967). *A theory of leadership effectiveness.* New York: McGraw-Hill.

House, R. H. (1971). A path-goal theory of leader effectiveness. *Administrative Science Quarterly, 16*, 321–338.

House, R. H. (1977). A 1976 theory of charismatic leadership. In J. Hunt & L. Larson (Eds.), *Leadership: The cutting edge.* (pp. 21–26). Carbondale, IL: Southern Illinois University Press.

Kelly-Heidenthal, P. (2003). *Nursing leadership & management.* Clifton Park, NY: Thomson Delmar Learning.

Kerr, S., & Jermier, J. (1978). Substitutes for leadership: Their meaning and measurement. *Organizational Behavior and Human Performance, 22*, 374–403.

Kirkpatrick, S. A., & Locke, E. A. (1991). Leadership: Do traits matter? *The Executive, 5*, 48–60.

Leach, L. S. (2003). Leadership and Management. In P. Kelly-Heidenthal (Ed.), *Nursing leadership & management* (pp. 157–179). Clifton Park, NY: Thomson Delmar Learning.

Lewin, K. (1939). Field theory and experiment in social psychology: Concepts and methods. *Journal of Sociology, 44*, 868–896.

Locke, E. A. (1968). Toward a theory of task motives and incentives. *Organizational Behavior and Human Performance, 3*, 157.

McCall, M. W., Jr. (1998). *High flyers: Developing the next generation of leaders.* Boston, MA: Harvard Business School Press.

Northouse, P. (2001). *Leadership: Theory and practice* (2nd ed.). Thousand Oaks, CA: Sage.

Rozier, C. K. (1996). Nurse executive characteristics: Gender differences. *Nursing Management, 27*(12), 33–37.

Rudan, V. T. (2003). The best of both worlds: A consideration of gender in team building. *Journal of Nursing Administration, 33*(3), 179–186.

Skinner, B. F. (1953). *Science and Human Behavior.* New York: Free Press.

Sullivan, E. J., & Decker, P. J. (2001). *Effective leadership and management in nursing* (5th ed.). Upper Saddle River, N.J.: Prentice Hall.

Wheatley, M. J. (1992). *Leadership and the new science: Learning about organization from an orderly universe.* San Francisco: Berrett-Koehler.

Additional Resources

Adams, J. S. (1963). Toward an understanding of inequity. *Journal of Abnormal and Social Psychology, 67*, 422.

Adams, J. S. (1965). Injustice in social exchange. In (Berkowitz, L.) *Advances in Experimental Social Psychology.* Vol. 2. New York: Academic Press.

Avolio, B. (1999). *Full leadership development: Building the vital forces in organizations.* Thousand Oaks, CA: Sage.

Bass, B. (1985). *Leadership and performance beyond expectations.* New York: Free Press.

Brandt, M. A. (1994). Caring leadership: Secret and path to success. *Nurse Manager, 25*(4), 68–72.

Burns, J. M. (1978). *Leadership.* New York: Harper & Row.

Cohen, S. (2004). Manager's fast track: Beam up staff with technology-savvy leadership. *Nursing Management, 35*(2), 12.

Conger, J., & Kanungo, R. (1987). Toward a behavioral theory of charismatic leadership in organizational settings. *Academy of Management Review, 12*, 637–647.

Goleman, D. (1995). *Emotional intelligence.* New York: Bantam.

Laurent, C. L. (2000). A nursing theory for nursing leadership. *Journal of Nursing Management, 8*(2), 83–87.

Lussier, R. N., & Achua, C. F. (2001). *Leadership: Theory, application, skill development.* Cincinnati, OH: South-Western College.

McDaniel, C. (1992). Transformational leadership in nursing service: A test of theory. *Journal of Nursing Administration, 22*(2), 60–65.

Mitchell, T. R. (1974). Expectancy models of job satisfaction, occupational preference, and effort: A theoretical, methodological and empirical appraisal. *Psychological Bulletin, 81*, 1096.

Moorhead, G., & Griffin, R. W. (2001). *Organizational behavior: Managing people in organizations* (6th ed.). Boston, MA: Houghton-Mifflin.

Namerof, R. E., Abrams, M., & Ott, B. (2004). Building a nursing leadership infrastructure. *Nurse Leader, 2*(1), 33–37.

Nelson, J. L., Apenhorst, D. K., Carter, L. C., Mahlum, E., K., & Schneider, J. V. (2004). Professional issues: Coaching for competence. *MedSurg Nursing, 13*(1), 32–35.

Perkins, V. J. (1992). A model for selecting leadership styles. *Occupational Therapy and Health Care, 8*(2-3), 225–237.

Powell, G. N. (1999). *Handbook of gender and work.* Thousand Oaks, CA: Sage.

Rajotte, C. A. (1996). Empowerment as a leadership theory. *Kansas Nurse, 71*(1), 1.

Stodgill, R. M. (1974). *Handbook of leadership: A survey of theory and research.* New York: Free Press.

Web Sites

Advancing Women in Leadership online journal
http://www.advancingwomen.com/awl/awl.html

Archives of Nursing Leadership
   http://www.lib.uconn.edu/online/research/speclib/ASC/nursing/
   nursbroc.htm

Center for Leadership and Change Management (Wharton School, University of
Pennsylvania)
   http://leadership.wharton.upenn.edu/welcome/index.shtml

Healthcare Leadership Council
   http://www.hlc.org

Canadian Journal of Nursing Leadership
   http://www.nursingleadership.net

NHS National Nursing Leadership Project (UK)
   http://www.modern.nhs.uk/home/default.asp?site_id=58&id=1115

Nursing Leadership Forum
   http://www.springerjournals.com/store/home_nlf.html

CHAPTER

2

WHAT IS MANAGEMENT?

INTRODUCTION

Management, sometimes also referred to as supervision, is a complex process of coordinating, directing, and assigning both physical and human resources in order to accomplish an organization's short-term and long-term objectives. Effective management is achieved through six key functions (planning, staffing, organizing, directing, controlling, and decision making), and is impacted by a variety of organizational and people-centered characteristics. There is no consensus on how management actually *works*, but in the past 200 years, a variety of theories have been developed that attempt to explain management's complexities.

KEY POINTS

1. What is management?

   A. **Management** is the process of

      i. coordinating actions
     ii. directing actions
    iii. assigning resources

   B. The purpose of management is to perform these tasks in order to achieve the **objectives** (desired outcomes) of an organization.

   C. The terms management and **supervision** sometimes are used interchangeably; however, management is a broader concept that includes supervising people as well as using other resources to accomplish organizational goals.

   D. Management often focuses on issues such as costs, productivity, staffing, and effectiveness.

   E. These management issues may or may not have anything to do with leadership. Management does not equal leadership, although leadership may play a role in management.

      i. management is often synonymous with constant activity and interaction
     ii. in the course of a typical day, managers, usually, deal with many activities ranging from highly prioritized and crucial to routine (for example, from a downsizing decision that will send a nurse to a different unit, to making sure that a nurse's employment anniversary is recognized)
    iii. the most common image of a manager is of a "firefighter" who responds to problems that emerge randomly, and are addressed in order of urgency
    iv. most managers spend much of their time interacting with others (McCall, Morrison, & Hanman, 1978; Leach, 2003)

   F. Management functions consist of:

      i. **planning:** determining the objectives of an institution or organization and what needs to be done (both in the short term and long term) to achieve those objectives. According to Sullivan and Decker (2001), planning very often addresses the organizational questions of what, why, where, when, how, and by whom, and it usually consists of a four-stage process:
        a. establish objectives
        b. evaluate the present and predict future trends and events
        c. formulate a planning statement
        d. convert the plan into an action statement

    ii. **staffing:** selecting the people who are able to carry out the action plan. This selection is usually based on:
      a. the knowledge, skills, and experience of the nurse
      b. the number and type(s) of patients needing care
      c. number and type of support staff available (Leach, 2003)
   iii. **organizing:** based on the plan as well as knowledge about the structure of the institution or organization, organizing is the process of coordinating human and other resources to meet established goals. Effective organizing consists of
      a. knowledge of factors such as institution, environment, social structure, people, and technology
      b. ability to assign tasks appropriately to people who can accomplish the tasks successfully (delegation)
      c. coordinating tasks that have been assigned and changing tasks or staff if goals are not being met
      d. using appropriate and accepted types of authority to ensure that required tasks are completed. Depending on the organization and the manager, authority may derive from the manager's position in the organization itself, or from the relationship between supervisor and staff member (Sullivan & Decker, 1992, 2001). For example, in a more rigid organizational structure such as a police or fire department, authority comes with rank.
   iv. **directing:** motivating and leading personnel to accomplish objectives. How a person directs others depends on that person's authority, power, and leadership style. Effective directing is achieved through strategies such as:
      a. setting specific, clear expectations that are realistic and measurable
      b. providing sufficient resources to accomplish the tasks
      c. fostering a work environment that balances challenge and success
      d. finding ways to recognize and reward work that meets or exceeds objectives in a way that is meaningful to workers (Costello-Nickitas, 1997; Sullivan & Decker, 2001).
    v. **controlling:** establishing standards of performance, comparing results with these benchmarks, and correcting performance that differs from accepted standard. Frequently used means of control include:
      a. **management by objectives (MBO)** devices: determining objectives, measuring to see if objectives are being met, and comparing objectives with standards (benchmarks)
      b. **socialization:** often a key part of MBO, socialization means that nurses internalize professional values and standard codes of behavior. For nurses, socialization is a process of moving

from the early stages of accepting perceived beliefs and values of the profession, through formal and informal education, to the final stage of full membership in the profession and commitment to its norms and values (Sullivan & Decker, 1992).

   c. **managerial surveillance:** the direct observation of staff behavior by the manager as well as indirect observation, for example, through the manager's review of records. A key concept of this function is "span of control," which refers to the number of individuals for whom a supervisor is directly responsible. A **narrow span of control** means fewer numbers of directly supervised staff and thus higher degrees of direct observation and control. A wider span of control (more than 10 supervised employees) means less opportunity for direct observation or control. A **wide span of control** can be effective as long as staff members are highly educated, tasks are relatively routine, and managers can effectively oversee such a group (Van Fleet & Bedeian, 1977, Sullivan & Decker, 1992).

   d. **continuous quality improvement (CQI):** in this formal quality improvement process, staff members participate in and lead the team. All team members are continuously involved in peer review, so that they can identify ways to improve processes or programs, and constantly enhance and improve the quality of care (Sullivan & Decker, 2001).

  vi. **decision making:** key steps of this function include:
    a. identifying problems
    b. establishing criteria that can evaluate potential solutions to the problem(s)
    c. seeking alternative solutions, including taking no action
    d. evaluating all the alternatives that have been found
    e. selecting the best alternative, based on organizational objectives, staff, environment, and other available resources. (Sullivan & Decker, 2001, also see Chapter 8 for more information on decision making)

G. A variety of factors affect management roles and decisions. They include:

  i. the institution's structure (for example, size—how it handles authority, department size and structure, wide or narrow span of control, amount of centralization or decentralization, how it measures and controls outcomes, and how it selects, recruits, and rewards employees)

  ii. the organization's objectives: the service(s) it offers (such as a hospital that specializes in cardiology or an outpatient surgical center that specializes in cataract surgery), how productive the organization is or how efficiently it meets objectives, the quality

and amount of its human resources, and how employees participate in goal setting

iii. environmental factors (for example, the current economic, legal,
technological, or social influences that the organization must
consider)

iv. technology (for example, current state of medical or nursing science, process technology, computer systems, and informatics)

v. tasks that are required or expected (for example, the nature of
tasks that need to be completed, how work tasks are designed,
and the impact of the organization's physical layout on the
nature and design of tasks)

vi. social structure (for example, the organization's internal culture,
how it socializes employees, the rituals that it uses to conduct
work or deal with conflict, perceptions of authority, and language
and cultural issues) (Sullivan & Decker, 1992)

2. Current management theories. The modern era of management theory
began in the 1800s with the Industrial Revolution and the widespread
development of factory work. Following is a brief history of management
theory as well as the most frequently cited current theories.

A. **Scientific management**

i. established by engineer Frederick Taylor (*Principles of Scientific
Management*, 1911) but still in use

ii. focused on maximizing worker production levels and efficiency

iii. relied on the view of work as systematic series of tasks that
could be measured, predicted, and manipulated to increase
efficiency

iv. developed **time and motion studies** that resulted in "one best
way" of carrying out a specific task or series of tasks

v. one important medical application: this method revolutionized
the field of surgery (Gilbreth, 1912), as efficient surgical methods resulted in shorter operations and reduced risks to
patients

vi. this approach can also provide important feedback about work-
flow; where equipment, medications, and other items essential
for patient care are stored and how they can be positioned to
enhance nursing efficiency (so nurses don't waste time walking
long distances to supply closets, for example)

B. **Bureaucratic theory**

i. developed by Max Weber.

ii. in contrast to the traditional European family-type organizational
structure in which employees are loyal to an individual manager

or supervisor, Weber argued that efficiency is achieved through impersonal relations within a formal structure (bureaucracy)

   iii. focused on employee competence as the basis for hiring and promoting employees (rather than interpersonal relationships with superiors)

   iv. emphasized the orderly and rational, not the interpersonal

   v. promoted strong top-down hierarchy with clear superior-subordinate communication and relationships. In this model, a person's power is assigned, based on the authority of his rank or position.

C. **Administrative theory**

   i. originally developed by French mining engineer Henri Fayol (1916)

   ii. states that several principles are essential to the functioning of any organization: planning, organizing, coordinating, and controlling

   iii. additional component of management process is unity of command and direction (workers get orders from only one supervisor and related work tasks are grouped under one manager)

   iv. theory also recognizes the power of the informal structure in organizations (Barnard, 1938), which identifies the role of naturally forming social groups and the recognition that they are powerful forces in organizations

   v. Barnard believed that managers must recognize and work with these informal structures to achieve the best outcomes for the organization

D. **Human relations theory** (later called organizational behavior)

   i. focuses on the individual worker—rather than processes and procedures—as the key to organizational motivation, productivity, and control

   ii. studies in the 1930s showed that workers are motivated by other workers as much as by environmental factors

   iii. the **Hawthorne effect,** which was identified during these studies, says that when a person is observed or studied, his or her behavior changes (Hughes, Ginnett, & Curphy, 1999, Leach, 2003)

E. **Motivational theory.** This group of theories grew out of human relations theory, which emphasized that worker output was best when workers were treated humanely. According to the motivation theory:

   i. motivation is interpreted from people's behavior rather than explicitly demonstrated by their actions

   ii. motivation is an internal process that directs behavior to satisfy needs

      iii. understanding motivation is the key because it helps explain why people do what they do; understanding workers' motivation can help managers create change

      iv. most well-known motivation theories are those based on:

        a. Maslow's (1970) hierarchy of needs (physical needs must be satisfied before higher psychological needs)

        b. Herzberg's (1968) theory (maintenance factors include adequate wages and safe workplace; motivations include meaningful work, recognition of accomplishments, and development opportunities)

        c. McGregor's (1960) theory (Theory X: leaders must direct and control worker motivation and Theory Y: workers are self-controlled and self-disciplined and the leader's job is to remove obstacles from their work and help them meet their personal goals)

        d. Ouchi's (1981) theory (Theory Z: the best way to motivate is through collective decision making, long-term job security, use of quality circles, and humanistic management style) (Leach, 2003)

3. The changing world of nursing and management

    A. Management often derives from a more rigid, hierarchical structure. In traditional organizations:

      i. a manager is an expert in management techniques, but not necessarily an expert in clinical realm. This can lead to

        a. managers being targets of downsizing

        b. managers becoming overseers of systems (clinical, cost information, data) rather than of people. This means the manager has a vested interest in maintaining these systems even if redesign will be more efficient and will result in better patient outcomes.

      ii. the disengaged manager is not a model that works well in nursing

        a. nurses need clinical managers who have knowledge of the challenges bedside caregivers face so as to be able to support staff and advocate for staff needs to superiors

        b. nurses tend to be put off by managers who could not participate in patient care if necessary during a crisis

    B. Ongoing dilemma for nursing: the combination of clinical and management skills

      i. expert clinicians are often promoted to nurse manager positions based on their clinical expertise, and not their management skills. In many organizations, this is the only opportunity for advancement

   ii. however, someone with great management skills may not be up-
        to-date clinically

C.   Management without leadership: According to S. Covey (1989, p.102),
     management without leadership is "like straightening deck chairs on
     the Titanic."

REVIEW ACTIVITIES

Questions

1. The purpose of management is to coordinate and direct actions and assign
    resources in order to.
    a. achieve the organization's objectives
    b. receive a promotion
    c. develop high quality staff
    d. keep staff turnover as low as possible

2. Which of the following statements about management is true?
    a. it focuses on clinical excellence
    b. it tends to attract people who like quiet, routine work without
        interruptions
    c. it focuses on issues such as cost, productivity, effectiveness, and
        staffing
    d. it is synonymous with leadership

3. The management function that involves determining the objectives of an
    organization and tasks needed to complete objectives is
    a. staffing
    b. directing
    c. planning
    d. controlling

4. When a person internalizes a set of standards or codes of behavior, this is
    called
    a. decision making
    b. managerial surveillance
    c. productivity
    d. socialization

5. A manager with a narrow span of control will
    a. directly supervise more than 10 staff members
    b. have greater opportunities for direct observation and control of staff

c.   tend to oversee staff with high levels of training
d.   be unable to motivate staff members

6. Identifying problems, establishing criteria, seeking and evaluating alterna-
    tives, and selecting the best choice are steps in the management function of:
    a.   controlling
    b.   decision making
    c.   staffing
    d.   directing

7. MBO stands for management by
    a.   organization
    b.   opposition
    c.   objectives
    d.   oversight

8. The time and motion studies developed by _____ resulted in
    "one best way" of carrying out a specific task.
    a.   Frederick Taylor
    b.   Max Weber
    c.   Henri Fayol
    d.   Abraham Maslow

9. According to bureaucratic theory, which of the following is true?
    a.   efficiency is achieved through personal relations between an employee
         and supervisor
    b.   there is no need for hierarchy, as all workers have a key role in the
         organization
    c.   employees should be hired based on their relationship with the
         owner
    d.   effective organizations are rational and orderly

10. Maslow, Herzberg, McGregor, and Ouchi developed theories about
    worker behavior, based on which school of thought?
    a.   scientific theory
    b.   motivational theory
    c.   administrative theory
    d.   socialization theory

Critical Thinking Questions

1. A nurse is working on a medical-surgical unit, and a physician has just
    given her an order to insert a Foley catheter into a patient and send a urine
    sample to the laboratory. The nurse manager has instructed her that it is

time to go off the unit for her lunch break; if she doesn't leave the unit now, she will not be able to take her meal break when the cafeteria is open. Apply your knowledge of administrative theory to describe the problem in this situation. Choose another theory of management that could be applied in this situation, and explain how it would help the nurse solve her dilemma.

2. A hospital is building a new medical-surgical unit as an addition to the building. Describe how scientific management theory can be used to help design the new unit to maximize nursing efficiency.

Discussion Questions

1. Based on your experience in organizations or institutions, what types of management theories seem to be at work?

2. Think about the most effective supervisor you have had (in nursing or another job). What functions discussed in this chapter did you observe this person performing?

3. If you could create a perfect manager, how would he or she function? You may base your answer on the management theories discussed in this chapter or create one of your own.

Works Cited

Barnard, C. (1938). *The functions of the executive*. Boston, MA: Harvard University Press.

Costello-Nickitas, D. (1997). *Quick reference to nursing leadership* Albany, NY: Thomson Delmar Learning.

Covey, S. (1989). *The seven habits of highly effective people*. New York: Simon and Schuster.

Fayol, H. (1916/1949). (C Storrs, Trans.). *General and industrial management*. London: Pittman.

Herzberg, F. (1968, January/February). One more time: How do you motivate employees? *Harvard Business Review*, 53–62.

Hughes, R. L., Ginnett, R. C., & Curphy, G. J. (1999). *Leadership: Enhancing the lessons of experience* (3rd ed.). San Francisco: Irwin McGraw-Hill.

Kelly-Heidenthal, P. (2003). *Nursing leadership & management*. Clifton Park, NY: Thomson Delmar Learning.

Leach, L. S.(2003). Leadership and management. In P. Kelly-Heidenthal (Ed.), *Nursing leadership & management* (pp. 157–179). Clifton Park, NY: Thomson Delmar Learning.

Maslow, A. (1970). *Motivation and personality* (2nd ed.). New York: Harper & Row.

McCall, M. W. Jr., Morrison, A. M., & Hanman, R. L. (1978). *Studies of managerial work: Results and methods* (Tech. Rep.) Greensboro, NC: Center for Creative Leadership.
McGregor, D. (1960). *The human side of enterprise.* New York: McGraw-Hill.
Ouchi, W. (1981). *Theory Z: How American business can meet the Japanese challenge.* Reading, MA: Addison-Wesley Publishing.
Sullivan, E. J. & Decker, P. J. (1992). *Effective management in nursing* (3rd ed.). Redwood City, CA: Addison-Wesley Publishing.
Sullivan, E. J., & Decker, P. J. (2001). *Effective leadership and management in nursing* (5th ed.). Upper Saddle River, N.J.: Prentice Hall.
Taylor, F. (1911). *Principles of scientific management.* New York: Harper & Row.
Van Fleet, D. D., & Bedeian, A. G. (1977). A history of the span of management. *Academy of Management Review, 2,* 364.

Additional Resources

Fraser, K. D., & Strange, V. (2004). Decision making and nurse case management: A philosophical perspective. *Advances in Nursing Science. 27*(1), 32–43.
Gilbreth, L. M. (1921). *The Psychology of Management,* New York: Macmillan.
Marriner-Tomey, A. (2000). *Guide to nursing management and leadership* (6th ed.). St. Louis, MO: Mosby.
Marquis, B. C., & Huston, C. J. (2000). *Leadership roles and management functions in nursing* (3rd ed.). Philadelphia: Lippincott Williams & Wilkins.
Sullivan, J., Bretschneider, J., & McCausland, M. P. (2003). Designing a leadership development program for nurse managers: An evidence-driven approach. *Journal of Nursing Administration, 33*(10), 544–549.
Tappen, R. M., Weiss, S. A., & Whitehead, D. K. (2002). *Essentials of nursing leadership and management* (3rd ed.). New York: F.A. Davis Co.
Young, J., Urden, L. D., Wellman, D. S., & Stoten, S. (2004). Management curriculum redesign: Integrating customer service expectations for new leaders. *Nurse Educator, 29*(1), 41–44.
Wooten, L. P., & Crane, P. (2003). Nurses as implementers of organizational culture. *Nursing Economics, 21*(6), 275–79.

Web Sites

Educational Psychology Interactive: Maslow from Valdosta State University
http://chiron.valdosta.edu/whuitt/col/regsys/maslow.html

International Council of Nurses Position Statement on Management of Nursing and Health Care Services
http://www.icn.ch/psmanagement00.htm

Internet Guide for Nursing Managers and Executives
http://www.pohly.com/admin_nurse.html

Journal of Nursing Management online
www.ingenta.com/journals/browse/bsc/jnm

Maslow's Hierarchy of Needs Related to Employee Motivation
http://www.accel-team.com/maslow_/index.html

Nursing Management (UK)
http://www.nursing-standard.co.uk/nursingmanagement

CHAPTER

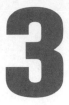

3

LEADERSHIP VERSUS MANAGEMENT

INTRODUCTION

Should nurses strive to be leaders or managers? In most organizations, leaders and managers are seen as having different roles, with leaders focusing on skills that help develop people and their abilities, while managers are more concerned with keeping the organization running as efficiently as possible. In the ever-changing world of health care today, most nurses will need both leadership and management skills.

KEY POINTS

1. Leadership and management:

   A. The two concepts are not interchangeable.

      i. Leaders do the right thing. Managers do things right (Bennis & Nanus, 1985).

      ii. Leaders get other people to want to do something, while managers get other people to do what they do not want to do (Kouzes & Posner, 1990).

      iii. Management works within the paradigm. Leadership creates new paradigms. Management works within the system. Leadership works on the system. You manage "things" but you lead "people" (Covey & Merrill, 1994, p. 27).

    iv. However, leadership and management do not have to work against one another, as these descriptions imply. Leaders can be effective managers and managers can be effective leaders.

B.   **Leadership** today is the preferred mode of "getting things done" in health care. According to Costello-Nickitas (1997), successful nurse leaders

    i. respond flexibly to changes in the workplace
    ii. disseminate information rapidly and effectively through their teams
    iii. develop and maintain strong trust and interpersonal connections with staff, peers, patients, and other health care professionals
    iv. build up and support team members' skills and strengths, while dealing effectively with differences
    v. do not avoid uncertainty or chaos but instead thrive on it

C.   Other characteristics of nurse leaders include:

    i. specialists and generalists: effective leaders are experts in a particular field. In nursing, for example, this specialization could be in emergency care or community health practice. Nurse leaders are also generalists; they know enough about a wide range of areas so that they are able to communicate with and mediate between a variety of other specialists and specialty practice areas.
    ii. self-reliance: effective nurse leaders understand that they must rely on themselves (to listen, make good decisions, maintain clinical skills, etc.) but they effectively balance this self-reliance against their value to and role within the organization
    iii. connectedness: effective nurse leaders are always excellent team players, and almost always key members of more than one team in an organization (Costello-Nickitas, 1997)

D.   Roles and functions of nursing managers. According to the American Organization of Nurse Executives (AONE, 1992), the nurse manager is accountable for:

    i. excellence in nursing clinical practice and delivery of patient care in a particular unit or area of an organization
    ii. managing human, monetary, and other resources needed to provide excellent patient care and achieve expected outcomes
    iii. facilitating the development of nursing and health care personnel (both licensed and unlicensed) in a designated unit or department
    iv. ensuring that all standards of care practiced in that area are in compliance with professional (Nurse Practice Act), regulatory (JCAHO), and government (local, state and federal) standards of care

    v. developing strategic planning that supports the department's or unit's and organization's overall mission

    vi. facilitating relationships among different departments or disciplines to ensure the delivery of the highest quality patient care

E. Key nurse **management** roles in the health care environment (note that organizations have different names for these functional roles):

    i. first-line manager: the **nurse manager** primarily supervises other nonmanagerial staff and monitors the quality of care that staff provide to patients. This manager is also responsible for motivating staff to meet organizational goals. The remainder of the nurse manager's time is usually spent in planning and coordination and staff evaluation. Key tasks that a first-line nurse manager may perform include:

      a. preparing orientation schedule in collaboration with nurse educators

      b. submitting time schedules for nursing shifts

      c. staff assignments for patient care during shifts

      d. making budget recommendations to nursing administration based on unit needs and patient acuity

      e. calculating amount of staff needed and meeting challenges when staff members call out sick, or other situations disrupt the staffing schedule

      f. making daily patient rounds

      g. conducting meetings with staff

      h. conducting employment reviews, including counseling reports and termination

      i. setting goals for individual patient care areas

      j. participating in quality assurance activities

      k. maintaining clinical knowledge through reading journals, participating in continuing education activities, and other opportunities for learning

    ii. middle-level manager: the **nurse director** supervises first-level managers, usually within a geographic or specialty area and is responsible for all people and activities in this area. The mid-level manager spends more time planning, coordinating, negotiating, and evaluating, and less time directly supervising staff. Increasingly, this level of responsibility requires graduate level education. Key tasks that a middle-level manager may perform include:

      a. assessment: observe whether policies and objectives are meeting the needs of patients and the staff that provide care

      b. planning: set short-term and long-term goals for patient care, revise policies if needed so that patient care objectives can be met and outcomes can be achieved most efficiently

      c. organization: put plans in action (via delegation and commit-
tee work) by developing appropriate teaching strategies, organizing budget to meet planning needs, engaging in customer
relations and communication to improve outcomes and manage risk effectively

      d. control: analyze results of implementation, consider changes
that need to be made, facilitate nurse managers in research
and development, and communicate changes and opportunities to managers and staff

  iii. executive-level manager: the **chief nurse executive** or **vice president of patient care services** spends the lowest amount of time in
supervision; most of the time is spent in planning and making policies. This person is less responsible for direct supervisory activities and more responsible for establishing overall organizational
goals and strategic plans for a department, division, or entire
organization—oversight often includes nonnursing areas. As with
the middle-level manager, the responsibilities for this position usually require significant managerial experience and graduate level
education (may be in business, in addition to or instead of nursing).
Key tasks that the nursing executive might perform include:

      a. assessment: understand the organization's internal environ-
ment or culture and the external environment (bioethics, legislation, regulation, technology, community) in which it must
function

      b. planning: forecast trends in health care, costs, reimbursement,
and regulation, and developing responsive strategic plans

      c. organization: based on assessment and strategic planning,
bring together the appropriate mix of staff, other resources,
ongoing research, and education

      d. control: evaluate nursing policies, programs, and services, to
ensure they are consistent with the organization's mission and
objectives and the needs of the patients and of the staff (Leach,
2003; Sullivan & Decker, 2001)

F. Other managerial roles that have evolved

  i. **charge nurse** (also called resource nurse)

      a. expanded staff nurse role with some managerial responsibility
on a given shift in a frontline role

      b. may be a permanent or rotating assignment

      c. usually functions as a liaison to the nurse manager, particularly
on off-shifts

      d. tasks include assisting in shift coordination, promoting quality
care, using resources efficiently, troubleshooting problems that
occur, and helping staff members with making decisions and
prioritizing care

        e. differs from first-level manager in that a charge nurse has more limited authority and limited scope of responsibility; depending on the organization, the charge nurse may or may not be involved in staff evaluations (may be more involved in off-shifts in which the manager has less direct observation of staff members)

    ii. **staff nurse**

        a. this position may not have formal managerial rank but the nurse uses managerial and leadership skills to work with other nurses and assistive personnel

        b. management responsibilities include supervising to ensure quality patient care, delegating tasks appropriately, and motivating staff (Sullivan & Decker, 2001)

G. **Mintzberg**'s (1994) contemporary model of managerial work says that managerial functions occur at three levels—information, people, and action.

    i. information processing: the most abstract level—including communicating (sharing) information with others as well as controlling (using information to manage others' work)

    ii. people: at this level, the manager leads (encourages and enables) people and links people (establishes networks) to help them be effective

    iii. action: at this level, the manager is very involved in "doing"—this includes supervisory actions such as directing change, handling disturbances, and negotiating

H. According to Costello-Nickitas, characteristics that distinguish leaders and managers include:

    i. facilitator vs. director: leaders provide their staff with resources that enable them to learn and solve problems, rather than giving directions on how tasks "should be" done

    ii. coordinating vs. controlling: effective leaders excel at stepping back and allowing people to use their own initiative to solve problems with some support, but minimal guidance. Leaders then are free to work at a higher level, coordinating a variety of able employees, rather than controlling or directing employees' every move.

    iii. pull vs. push: effective leaders encourage and motivate people to act rather than ordering them to act

    iv. macromanagement vs. micromanagement: effective leaders tend to look at the big picture, which involves standards and policies, rather than focusing on a series of tasks. Micromanagement is often perceived by staff as indicating that they are incompetent or not to be trusted to act appropriately when independent.

      v. peers/followers vs. subordinates: leaders tend to follow a less hierarchical approach to working with others, thus seeing staff members as part of a team rather than as located at higher or lower levels of an organization. This more open structure facilitates feedback and communication.

     vi. coaching/challenging vs. blaming: effective leaders use mistakes or problems as learning opportunities that provide a chance for coaching staff in proper procedures or challenging them to increase their level of competence or performance rather than blaming, chastising, or punishing.

    vii. solving problems vs. just identifying them: effective leaders are active problem solvers, balancing the various needs of staff and the organization, matching resources appropriately with problems, and promoting both efficiency and care in an environment that is focused on patient care (Costello-Nickitas, 1997). These leaders may see problem solving as so effortless that they are not aware they are doing it; a problem-solving approach simply seems natural to them.

2. In many organizations, leaders and managers have very different roles:

  A. Leadership

      i. key role is prioritizing and optimizing patient care

     ii. focus is first on patient outcomes and then on "bottom line" outcomes

  B. Management

      i. priority is the function of the organization

     ii. particular focus on meeting financial or business goals

3. Difference in the two concepts tends to be emphasized by current health care financial setting.

  A. Impacts on leadership

      i. figuring out how to care for high acuity patients with fewer resources

     ii. keeping staff together as a cohesive unit with a history that can build toward the future

    iii. helping integrate intrinsic rewards of nursing into the work

  B. Impacts on management

      i. providing care is a continuum both inside the institution and in the community, rather than a series of isolated service departments or individual organizations

     ii. organizations tend to become more consolidated and maybe managed from a central location

     iii. organizations (and people within them) will be required to form a variety of partnerships, both inside and outside the organization (Carroll, 1998)

     iv. mergers and acquisitions can change organizational culture, alter expectations, create fears about job security, and cause upheaval in day-to-day operations

C.   Leadership principles can be more difficult to implement in the strongly hierarchical and inflexible corporate structure of health care facilities. However, leadership principles will become increasingly necessary for this environment to function effectively.

REVIEW ACTIVITIES

Questions

1. Which of the following is a characteristic of an effective nurse leader?
   a.   following rules precisely
   b.   developing strong and trusting relationships with staff
   c.   withholding strategic information for long periods of time
   d.   focusing on the business of health care

2. A nurse manager who spends 90% of his or her time submitting time schedules for nursing shifts and assigning teams and patients is at what level of management?
   a.   first-line nurse manager
   b.   middle-level manager
   c.   chief nurse executive
   d.   vice president of patient care services

3. The advantage of a nurse leader being both a generalist and a specialist is that the nurse can:
   a.   delegate all tasks to others
   b.   operate effectively without input from other staff members
   c.   choose not to be part of a management team
   d.   be an expert on a topic as well as communicate with a variety of other specialists

4. Which of the following is true about the nurse leader's trait of self-reliance?
   a.   It prevents the nurse leader from working effectively in a team.
   b.   It is a characteristic only of nurse managers, not of nurse leaders.

    c. It balances the nurse's personal abilities with the needs of the organization.

    d. It allows the nurse leader to accomplish multiple tasks without any assistance.

5. A focus on meeting an organization's financial or business goals is a function of:

    a management

    b. leadership

    c. problem solving

    d. coaching

6. The level of nursing manager that spends the least time directly supervising certified and noncertified nursing staff is:

    a. nurse executive

    b. middle-level manager

    c. first-level manager

    d. charge nurse

7. A staff nurse with some increased managerial responsibilities is usually called a(n)

    a. nurse executive

    b. charge nurse

    c. nurse assistant

    d. associate director of nursing

8. According to Mintzberg's model of managerial work, effective managers:

    a. act first and then communicate

    b. are seldom involved in leading people or forming networks

    c. manage action by doing, for example, directing change or negotiating

    d. lead at the first level, act at the second level, and communicate in summary form

Critical-Thinking Questions

1. Nurse Amerone has been given responsibility for developing a new care model for a dedicated orthopedic inpatient unit in an acute care hospital. Besides a nursing staff, should other health care professionals be members of the staff for such a unit? If yes, how could others be integrated under an RN manager?

2. All of the beds in the emergency department have been filled for hours because half of the beds are occupied by patients who have been admitted and are waiting to go to their beds upstairs. The nurses in the ED are angry at nurses working in the medical-surgical units, the ICU, the

CCU, and the telemetry unit for not taking the patients. For each level of nurse manager (charge nurse, nurse manager, nurse director, and nurse executive) describe how this problem would be addressed based on role performance.

Discussion Questions

1. In your own words, explain the difference between leadership and management. Do you know someone who is more of a manager than a leader or more a leader than a manager?
2. Interview a hospital-based nurse educator. Does someone in this role function as both a leader and a manager? Is one role more important than the other in order to be successful as an educator?

Works Cited

American Organization of Nurse Executives (1992). The role and function of the hospital nurse executive. In *American Hospital Association Advisory*. Chicago: American Hospital Association.

Bennis, W., & Nanus, B. (1985). *Leaders*. New York: Harper & Row.

Carroll, P. (1998). *The surgical nurse's managed care manual*. Boston, MA: Total Learning Concepts.

Costello-Nickitas, D. (1997). *Quick reference to nursing leadership* Albany, NY: Thomson Delmar Learning.

Covey, S., & Merrill, R. (1994). *First things first*. New York: Simon & Schuster.

Kouzes, J., & Posner, B. (1990). *The leadership challenge*. San Francisco: Jossey-Bass.

Leach, L. S. (2003). Leadership and management. In P. Kelly-Heidenthal (Ed.), *Nursing leadership & management* (pp. 157–179). Clifton Park, NY: Thomson Delmar Learning.

Mintzberg, H. (1994). Managing as blended care. *Journal of Nursing Administration, 24,* 29–36.

Sullivan, E. J., & Decker, P. J. (1992). *Effective management in nursing* (3rd ed.). Redwood City, CA: Addison-Wesley Publishing.

Sullivan, E. J., & Decker, P. J. (2001). *Effective leadership and management in nursing* (5th ed.). Upper Saddle River, N.J.: Prentice Hall.

Additional Resources

Marriner-Tomey, A. (2000). *Guide to nursing management and leadership* (6th ed.). St. Louis, MO: Mosby.

Marquis, B. C., & Huston, C. J. (2000). *Leadership roles and management functions in nursing* (3rd ed.). Philadelphia: Lippincott Williams & Wilkins.

Tappen, R. M., Weiss, S. A., & Whitehead, D. K. (2002). *Essentials of nursing leadership and management* (3rd ed.). New York: F.A. Davis Co.

Young, J., Urden, L. D., Wellman, D. S., & Stoten, S. (2004). Management curriculum redesign: Integrating customer expectations for new leaders. *Nurse Educator, 29*(1), 41–44.

Web Sites

American Organization of Nurse Executives
http://www.hospitalconnect.com/aone/about/home.html

Internet Guide for Nursing Managers and Executives
http://www.pohly.com/admin_nurse.htm

Leadership
http://www.1000ventures.com/business_guide/crosscuttings/leadership_main.htm

Leadership Development (leadership vs. management)
http://www.step-up-to-success.org/Leadership_Development2.html

Leadership vs. Management
http://www.1000ventures.com/business_guide/crosscuttings/leadership_vs_mgmt.html

CHAPTER

4

A POSITIVE DEFINITION OF POWER

charismatic power

coercive power

connection power

empowerment

expertise

group power

individual power

influence

information power

leadership

legitimacy

organizational power

politics

power

principle-centered power

punishment power

referent power

reward power

vision

INTRODUCTION

Power is defined as the ability or capacity to act. However, in the minds of many people, this word elicits images of control and coercion—the concept of "power over." This chapter discusses the role of positive power ("power with") as a key component of nursing leadership and as necessary for the empowerment of leaders and staff.

KEY POINTS

1. Definitions of Power

A. Having **power** means being able to make change, or to prevent change from happening. According to Miller (2003), for nurses, a positive definition of power means the ability to

     i. take resources by either creating them or acquiring them and

    ii. use them to meet goals such as providing safe and competent care as well as meeting organizational goals

B.   Bennis and Nanus (1985) note that "power has the energy to initiate and sustain action translating intention into reality, the quality without which leaders cannot lead" (p. 15).

C.   Stephen Covey (1990) says that power is the ability to act, the strength and potency to accomplish something. It is the vital energy to make choices and decisions. It is also the ability to overcome deeply embedded habits and to cultivate higher, more effective and productive habits.

D.   According to Costello-Nickitas (1997), **leadership** cannot exist without power.

E.   Power does not depend on the level at which a person sits in a hierarchy, but rather on "how an individual perceives power, how others perceive the individual, and the extent to which an individual can influence events" (Miller, 2003, p. 348).

F.   The concept of power in nursing is closely linked with **expertise**:

     i. expertise is validated through the nurse's skills and knowledge displayed in practice settings

    ii. nurses who believe they have the skills to influence events have a greater sense of their own power

G.   A positive definition of power emphasizes "power with" rather than "power over."

      i. "power with" style is available to all people, both leaders and nonleaders

     ii. this type of leadership focuses on a more democratic or participatory style

    iii. there is more emphasis on the influence of communication

    iv. decisions and policies reflect collaboration rather than coercion

     v. nurse leaders do need to be aware that some people in organizations prefer to use "power over" strategies that are designed to make the recipient feel incompetent, insecure, embarrassed, or forced to choose between limited (and unrealistic) options. As Sullivan and Decker (2001) note, nurses should be aware of these power plays and avoid responding to them.

H.   People achieve power through **influence**:

     i. according to Costello-Nickitas (1997), influence is "a skill used to gain power in interpersonal situations" (p. 32)

    ii. a person who can influence (help change) another person's feelings, attitudes, or behavior is powerful

2. Positive sources of power. Where does positive power come from? According to Fisher and Koch (1996), the key sources of power are the factors that help a person influence others to do what that person wishes. More specifically, according to Wells (1998), most nurses are able to exert influence through using one or more of the following:

A. **Expertise**

    i. skills and abilities the nurse possesses (can be clinical skills, communication skills, and problem-solving skills)

    ii. knowledge the nurse possesses. This generally focuses more on clinical knowledge but can also include knowledge about information systems, political structures, sources of data, available opportunities, and other knowledge (Fisher & Koch, 1996; Miller, 2003).

B. Legitimacy, or power derived from the position a nurse holds in a group. **Legitimacy** equates with degree of authority.

    i. focuses on personal authority that the nurse holds rather than authority designated by an organization

    ii. the group recognizes legitimate leaders and generally follows those with whom the group members agree. Leaders with whom the group significantly disagrees often lose their legitimacy.

    iii. legitimacy as the sole source of a person's power may not be sufficient in some settings, and may not be recognized in others (Fisher & Koch, 1996; Miller, 2003). For example, a nursing administrator without an educational background equal or higher than her contemporaries in other departments may not be perceived as having legitimate power. A nurse who is seen as legitimate in one setting or culture may not be seen in the same way in another setting; for example, a nurse who is an administrator in a small long-term care facility may not make an automatic transition to the same administrative position in a medium-sized community hospital. Men in nursing have struggled to achieve legitimacy in a predominantly female profession.

C. Admiration and trust, sometimes called **referent power** or **charismatic power**. This type of power is characterized by:

    i. a high level of respect for and trust in the charismatic individual

    ii. a significant amount of loyalty to the person who possesses referent power

This can explain the fact that followers sometimes rationalize or try to "explain away" any of the leader's behavior that is inconsistent.

    iii. a high level of confidence in followers, which depends on the trust in the charismatic leader. A leader with charismatic or referent power can be extremely influential, especially in difficult or stressful times (Fisher & Koch, 1996; Miller, 2003). However, this power can be easily abused. Franklin D. Roosevelt and John F. Kennedy are considered charismatic leaders, as were Charles Manson and David Koresh.

iv.   Among the most important characteristics of ethical charismatic leaders is the ability to develop creative, critical thinking in their followers and to stimulate followers to think independently and to question the leader's view to reduce the risk of blind loyalty that may ultimately be harmful to followers.

D.   **Information power**. According to Bower (2000), this type of leader characteristically

i.   has significant knowledge or understanding that is useful, accurate, or timely

ii.   readily shares this knowledge with others

iii.   does not rely on the organization to bestow power; the power comes from the person's own internal know-how and his or her willingness to share that power with others

iv.   must be recognized by the group as accurate and useful

E.   **Connection power**. The nurse leader who exercises this type of power, says Miller (2003), is aware that:

i.   all people are connected in some way to all other people. This is especially true in health care organizations and nursing communities in which people are connected through schools, professional organizations, and community affiliations. Everyone knows someone, who knows someone else . . . and so on.

ii.   people are attracted to making connections to people with power or their associates. No one, in nursing or elsewhere, likes to feel detached from sources of influence. Leaders who effectively exercise this type of power constantly remind themselves of people's need for connection and act in a way to foster those connections. For nurse leaders, this can be as simple as a verbal recognition of staff excellence or as complex as an award banquet.

iii.   people at all levels of an organization are connected, and those connections must be acknowledged and respected. As Miller (2003) notes, effective leaders recognize, for example, that workers at all levels of an organization have a complex web of relationships with more and less powerful people. If you are disrespectful of the hospital vice president's clerical staff, you can easily damage any relationship with the vice president as well.

F.   Honesty, integrity, and ethical practice—also called **principle-centered power**—have these characteristics:

    i. based on principles of honor, respect, loyalty, honesty, and integrity

   ii. how leaders choose what to do in any situation is based on these principles; all decisions made are measured against these principles. According to Sullivan and Decker (2001), nurses must understand and select behaviors that are in accord with principle-centered leadership, including:

      a. getting to know people and learning what they want and need

      b. being open: to keeping others informed, and to use trust and respect instead of fear and suspicion

      c. knowing one's own values and visions

      d. increasing interpersonal skills such as listening and expressing ideas clearly

      e. using personal power to enable others

      f. increasing connections between people and enlarging one's own sphere of influence (p. 93)

      g. understanding that in order to "win"one does not have to "lose" and that a win-win outcome can be the key to building ongoing, successful relationships

G. Guidelines for using power positively in organizations. According to Yukl and Tabor (1983), the following are effective ways for using the different types of power discussed earlier.

    i. Expert power

      a. preserve credibility (for example, by avoiding speculation or careless discussions)

      b. stay up-to-date with technology and other changes that affect people's work

      c. act with confidence and decisiveness in crises

      d. show respect and avoid arrogance; avoid damaging people's self esteem

      e. show concern for the perspectives of all people at all organizational levels; attempt to show how changes minimize risk to people

   ii. Authority/legitimacy power

      a. ask, don't demand

      b. make sure staff understands directions or questions

      c. explain why you are asking for something to be done

      d. follow up to ensure compliance

  iii. Referent/charismatic power

      a. be considerate, show concern for people, treat people fairly, and defend their interests to supervisors or outsiders

      b. avoid expressing (verbally or in action) hostility, rejection, distrust, or indifference toward people

      c. make requests that are reasonable

      d. be a positive role model

      iv. Connection power
         a. use relationships correctly and appropriately
         b. avoid name dropping
         c. be ready to reciprocate—if someone does a favor for you, offer to return the favor in a spirit of give and take, not keeping score
         d. recognize that all connections have limits, and abide by them (adapted from Sullivan & Decker, 2001, Box 4-1, p. 46)

  H. Power plus vision. According to Sullivan & Decker (2003), true power resides not in aggressiveness or coercion but in "the ability to make a conscious choice" (p. 96).

      i. understanding and gaining power relies on identifying your **vision**—what you and others in your organization really need and/or desire
      ii. power influences choices, and choices affect behaviors and feelings. A clear vision unites power and choices by:
         a. building consensus
         b. identifying capabilities
         c. determining factors needed for success
         d. identifying resources: people, time, and money

  I. Power can be held or exercised by different entities. The usual division is between personal power (which is centered in an individual) and organizational power (the power or authority exercised by, for example, a hospital, company, professional group, etc.).

      i. **individual power**: usually consists of personal characteristics (interpersonal skills, knowledge, charisma, trust) that are accepted and recognized
      ii. **group power**: more than one individual with a common vision or goal; many perspectives generally have more perceived power than just one
      iii. **organizational power**: this power derives from the organization's ability to set policy, assign revenues, hire and fire, and give out rewards or punishments

3. Other (less positive) sources of power.

  A. **Punishment** or **coercive power**. Most experts recognize that the power to punish or give negative incentives (dock someone's pay, issue a reprimand, termination) is sometimes necessary, as these penalties can discourage certain behaviors. However, as Miller (2003) notes, this type of power is perceived as

      i. humiliating by the person on the receiving end of the coercive power and thus
      ii. much less desirable for use by people in authority positions

      iii. however, some people who enjoy holding power over others may actually enjoy using punishment or coercive power, just to show they can

B. **Reward power**. As with coercive power, there can be a positive side. Reward power can encourage certain behaviors, and people may be motivated by monetary and other reward systems. However, Miller (2003) states:

      i. rewards that are assigned and distributed unfairly can have the opposite effect
      ii. rewards do not provide long-term changes in behavior or attitudes
      iii. withholding rewards can produce resentments
      iv. rewards don't motivate as effectively or as consistently as a clear, unifying vision
      v. If reward power is used, the leader should remember to
          a. avoid overdoing incentives; emphasize the intrinsic reward of teamwork and loyalty instead
          b. reinforce actual behavior rather than future performance
          c. ensure rewards reflect total, not partial, performance
          d. recognize that monetary awards may be the least effective
          e. carefully match the reward to the person; a reward for a unit secretary that is valued and appreciated may not have value for a registered nurse on the same unit

4. Empowerment is defined as "the process by which we facilitate the participation of others in decision making and take action within an environment where there is equitable distribution of power" (Kelly & Joel, 1996, p. 420).

A. Empowerment is built:

      i. through a commitment to the well being of all concerned, from the lowest to the highest levels of an organization
      ii. by providing an atmosphere in which risk taking is valued and encouraged to lead to or provide insights
      iii. with flexibility to adapt to changing priorities, needs, and situations
      iv. from diversity
          a. in styles of thinking, communication, and problem solving
          b. in accepting and encouraging culturally different points of view
      v. with cooperation rather than competition
      vi. though the ability to compromise (finding as many win-win solutions as possible)
      vii. with empathy for patients, other staff, management, and people in the community

B. Empowerment is demonstrated through:

    i. an increased ability to solve problems creatively and effectively

    ii. improved communication

        a. between nurses and patients

        b. between nursing team members (RN, LPN, nurse's aides, unit secretaries, and other assistive personnel)

        c. between nurses and other health team members (respiratory, physical and occupational therapists; pharmacists; and physicians, for example)

        d. between nurses and management

        e. throughout the organization

        f. between the organization and the community through community outreach programs

    iii. Increased satisfaction with work, including less stress and lower levels of burnout

    iv. Improvements in people's

        a. levels of self-esteem

        b. ability to function with autonomy

        c. levels of accountability and responsibility

5. Accepting power and becoming politically savvy. According to Costello-Nickitas (1997), effective nurse leaders are aware of the "three Ps" of the workplace—power, politics, and policy—and that these three entities must be addressed together (see earlier mentioned text for more about power).

A. Organizational **politics**

    i. Politics occurs because

        a. there is competition for the allocation of scarce resources (time, money, people, supplies) and thus

        b. competition for who gets to make the decisions

    ii. Knowledge of the politics of an organization is essential for effective use of power.

    iii. Effective political behavior includes

        a. persuasive skills, including the ability to appeal to others' needs and interests

        b. effective communication skills

        c. ability to develop coalitions, often with people in different areas to work toward a common goal

        d. interpersonal skills (both within and outside the organization)

B. Are "office politics" always bad?

    i. No, they can be positive

a. understanding organizational politics allows the nurse leader to see the informal power in an organization and avoid mistakes that can hamper the leader's ability to get things done
b. working within an organization's political structure can get things done faster, in an informal way when time is of the essence
c. being "plugged in" to informal communication systems will help keep the nurse leader informed of facts and perceptions. Even if perceptions and conclusions are false, they represent reality for many members of the organization and should not be ignored
d. knowing the political lay of the land allows the nurse leader to turn individual agendas into common goals
e. office political structures help build professional networks that help get things done

REVIEW ACTIVITIES

Questions

1. A nurse who has power is able to
   a. make staff do anything the nurse wants
   b. make or prevent change
   c. avoid engaging in organizational politics
   d. avoid decision making

2. According to this author, power includes the capacity to culture more effective habits.
   a. Nicolo Machiavelli
   b. Warren Bennis
   c. Stephen Covey
   d. Eleanor Sullivan

3. A characteristic of a "power over" strategy is that it makes the receiver feel
   a. empowered
   b. collaborative
   c. incompetent
   d. secure

4. A nurse's clinical abilities, education, and knowledge of systems are part of the power source known as:
   a. legitimacy
   b. charisma

    c.   connection

    d.   expertise

5. The source of power known as "connection power" is best described as

    a.   power that equates with the degree of the nurse's personal or organizational authority

    b.   power that is based on people's respect for or trust in a particular person

    c.   power based on honor, respect, loyalty, and integrity

    d.   power that derives from an awareness of the networks that exist between people in an organization

6. Leaders who make all their decisions based on their own ethical values (honesty, integrity, respect, etc.) are engaged in what kind of power?

    a.   expertise

    b.   principle-centered

    c.   legitimacy

    d.   charisma

7. An effective use of reward power would include

    a.   giving bonuses for future performance

    b.   using money as the primary reward system

    c.   rewarding total performance

    d.   giving incentives every day

8. Preserving credibility, staying current with technology, and acting decisively in crises are positive ways of using what type of power?

    a.   expert

    b.   reward

    c.   authoritative

    d.   charismatic

9. A person who effectively uses connection power would

    a.   do a lot of name dropping to emphasize connections

    b.   continually return to the same people for favors to build a network

    c.   build a group of networks based on different affiliations

    d.   understand that reciprocity is unimportant

10. Which of the following is true about punishment or coercive power?

    a.   penalties do not change people's behaviors

    b.   people appreciate being the recipient of this type of power

    c.   this type of power can include docking a person's pay, reprimands, or termination

    d.   this type of power should never be used in an organization

11. Which of the following is true about empowerment?

    a.   it establishes an atmosphere that discourages risk taking

    b.   it is clearly preferred by managers in health care organizations

    c.   it allows flexibility to adapt to changing priorities, needs, and situations

    d.   it encourages competition over cooperation

12. Effective political behavior in an organization is characterized by the ability to

    a.   appeal to other people's needs and interests

    b.   delay decision making for as long as possible

    c.   avoid competing for resources

    d.   validate all information from the organization's "grapevine"

Critical Thinking Questions

1. Using your knowledge of the entities of power, describe the powers that interact between an organization and a collective bargaining unit that represents workers in the organization.

2. When patients are empowered, are they more independent? Does that threaten established lines of power between the patient and the nurse or between the patient and the physician? What are the benefits and downsides of patient empowerment?

Discussion Questions

1. Based on your experience in a workplace, how do you define power? What sources of power are you more likely to draw on?

2. Choose an organization in your community that you know well. In which ways do its leaders and staff draw on the different sources of power (expertise, legitimacy, charismatic, information, connection, principle-centered)? Are some more effective than others?

3. What has been your experience of coercive power? Was it effective?

4. What are the organizational politics in your school, workplace, or other organizations you are involved with?

Works Cited

Bennis, W., & Nanus, B. (1985). *Leaders*. New York: Harper & Row.

Bower, F. L. (2000). *Nurses taking the lead: Personal qualities of effective leadership*. Philadelphia: Saunders.

Costello-Nickitas, D. (1997). *Quick reference to nursing leadership*. Albany, NY: Thomson Delmar Learning.

Covey, S. (1990). *Principle-centered leadership*. New York: Simon & Schuster.

Fisher, J. L., & Koch, J. V. (1996). *Presidential leadership: Making a difference.* Phoenix, AZ: American Council on Education and the Oryx Press.

Kelly, L. Y., & Joel, L. A. (1996). *The nursing experience: Trends, challenges, and transitions* (3rd ed.). New York: McGraw-Hill.

Miller, T. W. (2003). Power. In P. Kelley-Heidenthal (Ed.), *Nursing leadership & management* (pp. 347–357). Clifton Park, NY: Thomson Delmar Learning.

Sullivan, E. J., & Decker, P. J. (2001). *Effective leadership and management in nursing* (5th ed.). Upper Saddle River, NJ: Prentice Hall.

Yukl, G. A., & Tabor, T. (1983, March/April). The effective use of managerial power. *Personnel, 60*(2), 37–44.

Wells, S. (1998). *Choosing the future: The power of strategic thinking.* Boston: Butterworth-Heinemann.

Additional Resources

Benner, P. (2001). *From novice to expert: Excellence and power in clinical nursing practice.* Menlo Park, CA: Addison-Wesley Publishing.

Cloke, K., & Goldsmith, J. (2002). *The end of management and the rise of organizational democracy.* San Francisco: Jossey-Bass.

Kuokkanen, L., & Katajisto, J. (2003). Promoting or impeding empowerment? Nurses' assessment of their work environment. *Journal of Nursing Administration, 33*(4), 209–215.

Marriner-Tomey, A. (2000). *Guide to nursing management and leadership* (6th ed.). St. Louis, MO: Mosby.

Mintzer, B. (2000). Proceed with vision power. *Nursing Management, 32*(12), 19.

Parse, R. R. (2004). Power in position. *Nursing Science Quarterly, 17*(2), 101.

Robinson-Walker, C. (1999). *Women and leadership in health care: The journey to authenticity and power.* San Francisco: Jossey-Bass.

Sieloff, C. L. (2004). Leadership behaviours that foster nursing group power. *Journal of Nursing Management, 12*(4), 246–252.

Smith, S., Garland, G., & Miller, D. (2001). Power sharing . . . clinical leadership development. *Nursing Standard, 15*(50), 59.

Upenieks, V. (2003). Nurse leaders' perceptions of what compromises successful leadership in today's acute inpatient environment. *Nursing Administration Quarterly, 27*(2), 140–153.

Web Sites

A Look at Power in Nursing
    http://southflorida.sun-sentinel.com/careers/vitalsigns/partfolder/
    xiv08powern.htm

Internet Guide for Nursing Managers and Executives
http://www.pohly.com/admin_nurse.html

Nursing Image = Nursing Power
http://www.reallifehealthcare.com/rlh/news/story/9499418p-10423376c.html

Nursing Informatics: Infusing Nurses with Power for the 21st Century
http://www.nursing-informatics.com/

Nursing Power
http://www.nursingpower.net/index2.html

ACCOUNTABILITY IN NURSING LEADERSHIP

accountability
case management
chain of command
community
constituents
consumer demand
government

patient
patient-focused care
primary nursing
professional organizations
responsibility
shared leadership

INTRODUCTION

Accountability and responsibility are key qualities for nurses and nurse leaders as they provide care for patients and act as members of teams, organizations, communities, and countries. This chapter defines accountability and explores its applications for the nurse leader.

KEY POINTS

1. Accountability

    A. Definitions

        i. **Accountability** means being responsible and liable for one's decisions and actions (Kelly-Heidenthal, 2003, Glossary).

        ii. **Responsibility** involves being reliable and dependable, and obliged to accomplish work and to perform at an acceptable level based on education and training (Marthaler, 2003).

      iii. Responsibility denotes an obligation to accomplish a task, while accountability is accepting ownership for the results of that task or action (Sullivan & Decker, 2001, p. 222).

      iv. Accountability has traditionally been considered a hallmark of health care professions. Nurses have a primary responsibility for defining and providing nursing care.

      v. According to Miller (2003b), accountability and direct **responsibility** for decisions and actions are inherent in the nurse's role, and this is considered the hallmark of professionalism.

      vi. Accountability also includes being responsible for one's affiliations such as joining professional organizations or a collective bargaining unit.

B.   A nurse leader is accountable to a variety of **constituents**:

      i. the **patient**. Accountability-based care is provided to patients by nurses who are able to report, explain, and justify their actions. In this case, accountability means working toward and achieving outcomes. According to Sellers (2003), this care is provided through:

        a. **primary nursing** in which one nurse is accountable for a patient's care from admission to developing of care plan, implementing that plan, and overseeing the patient's discharge

        b. **patient-focused care** in which the nurse assumes accountability to oversee coordination of all care activities required by patients, including resources from other areas or departments and with assistive personnel

        c. **case management** in which the nurse is accountable for coordinating high-quality care while conserving health care resources

In all care scenarios, nurses are accountable for exhibiting ethical behavior, providing competent care, demonstrating appropriate thinking and problem-solving skills, and practicing leadership as appropriate.

      ii. the nurse himself or herself. For example, nurse leaders need to be accountable to themselves for

        a. maintaining the appropriate clinical skills and technical or scientific knowledge in order to provide safe care

        b. being aware of quality-of-life issues (such as stress management, job safety, working too many consecutive hours) that can affect the ability to deliver safe and appropriate care

        c. understanding current health care dynamics (such as legal or financial issues) that affect the ability to deliver safe and appropriate care

      iii. the people the nurse works with. As part of a team, the nurse is accountable for

        a. helping to maintain the function of nursing and interdisciplinary teams,

       b. maintaining a safe and appropriate working environment, and

       c. providing opportunities for health care professionals to maintain or enhance their skills and abilities

   iv. the health care organization the nurse works for, by reporting for work as required, not calling in sick arbitrarily, and being honest about his or her own knowledge base and personal limitations.

   v. the **community**. According to the Pew Health Professions Commission report (O'Neil, 1998), nurses are accountable to the community in a variety of ways, including:

       a. partnering with communities to make public and individual health care decisions

       b. helping underserved populations receive access to needed medical or nursing care

       c. practicing and promoting community-based and preventive care

   vi. the professional organizations with which the nurse is affiliated, for example, nursing **professional organizations** and licensing boards. Nurses are accountable for

       a. adhering to codes of professional conduct established by these groups

       b. holding accountable any colleagues who do not adhere to these codes of conduct (for example, nurses have an obligation to report a colleague who is impaired by substance abuse)

   vii. the **government** agencies that regulate nursing and health care. Nurses are accountable for:

       a. providing care that balances the needs of people, communities, and society

       b. working for the continuous improvement of the health care system

       c. advocating for public policies that promote and protect public health (O'Neil, 1998)

2. Accountability and leadership.

   A. Accountability often involves **shared leadership**. According to Sullivan and Decker (2001), shared leadership is an organizational structure in which several individuals jointly hold responsibility for achieving the organization's goals.

   B. Shared leadership depends on

     i. strong relationships and communication

     ii. workforce that is highly educated, competent, and capable of taking on leadership roles (a staff of professional registered nurses, for example)

      iii. abilities and knowledge that emerge in relation to the current
needs of the organization (rather than a "one person with the
answer" model)

      iv. examples of shared leadership include self-directed work teams,
shared governance, and coleadership, which are commonplace in
nursing departments today

3. Other aspects of accountability

  A. **Consumer demand** for accountability. The American Nurses Association (1995) states, "The authority for the practice of nursing is based
on a social contract that acknowledges professional rights and responsibilities as well as mechanisms for public accountability" (quoted in
Miller, 2003a, p. 152). A wide variety of consumer stakeholders demand
accountability by nurses in a variety of settings:

      i. inside the organization: customers (patients) and other nurses

      ii. outside the organization: communities, governmental bodies, and
members of the legal profession

Accountability can become a serious issue for an organization and its
employees when the focus on being competitive or financially solvent over-
rides the focus on providing the best quality health care.

Perceived lack of accountability generally leads to litigation by patients
who are not satisfied with health care outcomes.

  B. Accountability and effective use of **chain of command**. According to
Morgan (2003)

      i. nurses caring for patients have a legal and professional responsi-
bility to discuss problems or ask questions about orders that are
not clear. Doing so may require nurses to go through the chain of
command.

      ii. invoking chain of command means moving up the administrative
ladder when a nurse feels that the patient's clinical needs are not
being addressed.

      iii. clear, well-defined chain of command allows nurses who have
identified a problem that they cannot resolve to present it to pro-
gressively higher levels of authority in the hierarchy. Invoking
chain of command could include, for example,

        a. informing the immediate supervisor about the problem and
expressing explicit concern about the problem

        b. if that person's response is not satisfactory, the nurse is respon-
sible for contacting the next level of supervisor up, and so on,
until the problem is satisfactorily addressed.

      iv. every communication or attempted communication with each per-
son in the chain of command must be clearly and specifically documented (the circumstance will determine if these communications

should be documented in the patient record, in an incident report, or on personal notes that may be used for reference): who was contacted, time contacted, what was said

v. nurses who do not follow chain of command appropriately, risk loss of job, license (or both) as well as possible legal action; state laws govern whether and to what extent nurses are protected by whistle-blower legislation (see Chapter 22)

(see also Chapter 20 for more information on accountability and delegation)

REVIEW ACTIVITIES

Questions

1. Accountability is best defined as

a. being reliable, dependable, and obliged to accomplish work at an acceptable level
b. justifying actions to supervisors
c. being responsible and liable for decisions and actions
d. knowing how to move up the chain of command

2. Which of the following is true about accountability?

a. it is a hallmark of the health care professions
b. it seldom involves legal liability
c. it is separate from achieving care objectives
d. it must involve shared leadership

3. For all care scenarios, nurses are accountable for all of the following, except

a. exhibiting ethical behavior
b. providing competent care
c. demonstrating intuitive thinking skills
d. practicing leadership

4. Nurses are accountable for maintaining quality-of-life issues such as stress management to which of the following constituents?

a. patients
b. government
c. community organizations
d. themselves

5. Nurses are accountable to the government agencies that regulate health care by

a. holding colleagues accountable for following codes of conduct
b. working for continuous improvement of the health care system

c. helping underserved populations access health care
d. providing ways for health care professionals to enhance their skills

6. An organizational structure in which several individuals jointly hold
    responsibility for achieving the organization's goals is called
    a. shared leadership
    b. hierarchy
    c. chain of command
    d. authority-responsibility matrix

7. Which of the following is true about an organization's chain of command?
    a. It allows nurses to question orders and consult with the hierarchy of
        the organization
    b. It is used only for nursing issues and does not apply to physicians
    c. It prevents nurses from moving more than one level above the nurse's
        level of employment
    d. It does not require that the nurse reveal specific patient information

Critical-Thinking Questions

1. What does your state Nurse Practice Act say about each nurse's require-
    ments for reporting colleagues who do not follow the law?
2. What are your options for intervention if you are working with a nurse col-
    league who returns from a break with the odor of alcohol on her breath?
3. Describe how these principles of accountability and responsibility apply
    when a nurse makes a medication error that results in no harm to the
    patient.

Discussion Questions

1. In your own work, what does "being accountable" mean? How it is differ-
    ent from being "responsible"?
2. Think of an organization in your community. What are the responsibilities
    of its staff members? How are they accountable? To whom are they
    accountable? What happens if people are not responsible?
3. In health care organizations that you know, what most strongly drives
    accountability in that organization? Leaders inside the organization? Con-
    sumers of the product or service? Regulatory authorities?
4. Based on your experience, what are the most effective ways to promote
    responsibility and accountability in a health care organization?

Works Cited

American Nurses Association (1995). *Nursing's social policy statement.* Washington, DC: American Nurses Publishing. Cited in Miller, T. W. (2003a).

Kelly-Heidenthal, P. (2003). *Nursing leadership & management.* Clifton Park, NY: Thomson Delmar Learning.

Kelly-Heidenthal, P. (2003). America's health care environment. In P. Kelly-Heidenthal (Ed.), *Nursing leadership & management.* (pp. 1–31). Clifton Park, NY: Thomson Delmar Learning.

Marthaler, M. T. (2003). Delegation of nursing care. In P. Kelly-Heidenthal (Ed.), *Nursing leadership & management* (pp. 266–279). Clifton Park, NY: Thomson Delmar Learning.

Miller, T.W. (2003a). Politics and consumer partnerships. In P. Kelly-Heidenthal (Ed.), *Nursing leadership & management* (pp. 140–156). Clifton Park, NY: Thomson Delmar Learning.

Miller, T. W. (2003b). Power. In P. Kelly-Heidenthal (Ed.), *Nursing leadership & management* (pp. 347–357). Clifton Park, NY: Thomson Delmar Learning.

Morgan, D. W. (June, 2003). Going up the chain of command. *RN 66*(6), 67–70.

Neil, E. H., and the Pew Professions Commission. (December, 1998). *Recreating health professional practice for a new century.* Pew Health Professions Commission, pp. 29–43.

Sellers, K. F. (2003). First-line patient care management. In P. Kelly-Heidenthal (Ed.), *Nursing leadership & management* (pp. 280–299). Clifton Park, NY: Thomson Delmar Learning.

Sullivan, E. J., & Decker, P. J. (2001). *Effective leadership and management in nursing* (5th ed.). Upper Saddle River, NJ: Prentice Hall.

Additional Resources

Doherty, C., & Hope, W. (2000). Shared governance—nurses making a difference. *Journal of Nursing Management, 8*(2), 77–82.

Feldman, H. R. (2004). Accountability: Where the rubber meets the road. *Nursing Leadership Forum, 8*(3), 86–87.

George, V., et al. (2002). Developing staff nurse shared leadership behavior in professional nursing practice. *Nursing Administration Quarterly, 26*(3), 44–60.

Gillis, A. J. (2003). Personal accountability. *Canadian Nurse, 99*(10), 34–35.

Kelly, J. (2004). Accountability and recent developments in nursing. *Dimensions of Critical Care Nursing, 23*(1), 31–38.

Kupperschmidt, B. R. (2004). Making a case for shared accountability. *Journal of Nursing Administration, 34*(3), 114–116.

Murchison, I., Nicols, T. S., & Hanson, R. (1982). *Legal accountability in the nursing process.* St. Louis, MO: Mosby.

Silva, M., & Ludwick, R. (2002). Ethical grounding for entry into practice: Respect, collaboration, and accountability. *Online Journal of Issues in Nursing*. Retrieved November 26, 2005, from http://www.nursingworld.org/ojin/ethicol/ethics_9.htm

Web Sites

Accountability and Autonomy: Scottish Executive Health Department
http://www.show.scot.nhs.uk/sehd/practicenursing/workshops/morning_workshops_8.htm

American Nurses Association
http://www.nursingworld.org

Arizona Nurses Association: Chain of Command
http://www.aznurse.org/default.asp?PageID=10000724

Framework for Nursing in General Practice
http://www.show.scot.nhs.uk/sehd/practicenursing/workshops/morning_workshops_8.htm

Journal of Nursing Risk Management
http://www.afip.org/Departments/legalmed/jnrm.html

Nurse's Duty to Intervene: Initiating Chain of Command
http://www.thedoctors.com/risk/general/practiceguidelines/j4242.asp

Online Journal of Issues in Nursing
http://www.nursingworld.org/ojin

Part II

Primary Skills for the Nursing Leader

CHAPTER

6

WHAT IS COMMUNICATION?

KEY TERMS

accuracy
auditory communication channel
body language
channels
cognitive management apparatus
communication
communication models
communication process
decision support systems
diagonal communication
direct communication
downward communication
executive information systems
external interference
feedback
formal
hospital information systems
informal
interaction

interference
internal interference
kinesthetic communication channel
lateral communication
message
nonverbal communication
nursing information systems
pace
receiver
sender
Targowski-Bowman model
tone
tools
upward communication
verbal communication
visual communication channel
vocabulary
word choice

INTRODUCTION

Communication is how people exchange information and ideas. Although it may seem like a simple back and forth, it is actually a complex activity, and can have both tremendous potential and problems. Communication is an essential skill for leaders, and this chapter provides information to help leaders understand, analyze, and use communication skills effectively.

KEY POINTS

1. Communication is the exchange of information or opinions. Communication is, by definition, interactive. It is also complex and affected by a variety of elements, including the setting, the people engaged in communication, and the type of communication.

   A.   The following elements of the **communication process** are based on Laswell's (1948) model and include:

      i. **sender:** the originator of the message. A nurse who initiates a conversation ("How are you feeling today, Mrs. Jones?") acts as the sender.

     ii. **message:** the verbal and nonverbal stimuli relayed by the sender and taken in by the receiver. The words "How are you today?" are the verbal message. The nurse might also send a nonverbal message, such as raising the eyebrows to indicate interest or concern or touching the patient on the shoulder.

    iii. **receiver:** the person who takes in the message from the sender and processes it. For the question "How are you today, Mrs. Jones?" the receiver of the message is Mrs. Jones. When Mrs. Jones answers, "Fine, thank you" she becomes the sender and the nurse becomes the receiver.

    iv. **feedback:** the new message that is generated by the receiver in response to the original message by the sender. "How are you today, Mrs. Jones?" is the message from the nurse (sender) to Mrs. Jones (receiver). When Mrs. Jones says, "Fine, thank you," she is sending feedback to the nurse.

Feedback is considered effective when the two communicators understand each other's message and are able to shift roles appropriately between the sender and the receiver to exchange information or opinions (Ruthman, 2003).

   B.   Sullivan and Decker (1992) note five principles of effective communication:

      i. giving information is not the same as communication, which requires interaction, understanding, and response. For example, if a nurse asks a patient to do something, but the patient does not understand, information has been given but communication has not occurred.

     ii. sender is responsible for clarity. Nurse leaders must make sure that messages are clear—it is the leader's job to send understandable messages, not the receiver's job to "translate." When the receiver must translate, the sender runs the risk of the translation being different from the intended message.

      iii. use simple, exact language. The sender needs to use words that are precise and unambiguous so that the receiver is not confused.

      iv. communication encourages feedback. Although feedback is not always positive, it is essential for making sure that the receiver understands the message. Without feedback, the message may not be delivered. Feedback can be verbal ("I don't understand that") or nonverbal (such as a confused look, rolled eyes, or inability to follow directions given).

      v. senders must have credibility. A credible sender is perceived as trustworthy and reliable. Receivers who think the sender is not reliable may ignore the message.

      vi. use direct communication channels when possible. **Direct communication** (person-to-person, either face-to-face or in writing) is best because there is less chance of the message being distorted as it passes through different senders. Face to face direct communication is the most preferred as it allows the sender to get immediate feedback about the message.

B. The role of interference and interaction on communication elements. According to Lucas (2004),

      i. **Interference** is anything that impedes the communication of a message. For example, having your cell phone fade in and out is interference because it prevents the phone conversation from getting through. Or perhaps you are having a conversation with a patient and people on the other side of the curtain in the room are talking or laughing loudly. That is another example of interference. There are two types of interference:

          a. **external.** This type of interference originates outside a person, such as the earlier example. External interference can also include distractions such as having a television blaring. The result is that the receiver is distracted and the sender's message may not be fully received. Note that some people are more distracted by some types of external interference than others. For example, some people can "tune out" noise but others are completely distracted by it.

          b. **internal.** This type of interference comes from within the receiver. It can be physical (a headache, an itchy rash, a need to use the restroom, fatigue), or psychological (the receiver is concerned about being away from work, or worried about test results, or angry after a disagreement with a visitor).

      ii. **Interaction** of communication elements. The key to understanding the communication process is to know that

          a. all these elements (sender, receiver, message, feedback) have a distinct function

          b. each component interacts with other components

For example, a nurse tells a patient about a procedure (sender and message). The patient (receiver) provides feedback that he does not understand the preparation for the procedure. The nurse asks for more feedback, and understands that the patient does not understand some words. The nurse simplifies the vocabulary and then repeats the message. While repeating, the nurse notes that the patient seems distracted by the noise coming from a fire engine passing by outside. The nurse stops, begins the message again, and repeats it. The patient provides more feedback, this time about the timing of the procedure. The nurse waits until a second fire truck passes by, gives the information again, and follows up by handing the patient a list of written instructions that have a number of illustrations to enhance understanding.

C.   Communication **channels.** A communication channel is the means by which a message is communicated (Lucas, 2004). In the earlier example, the written instructions given to the patient are a communication channel. Communication channels are often categorized by one of the five senses that are used to process them. According to Ruthman (2003), there are three main channels of communication:

   i.   **visual.** For visual communication channels, receivers use sight to process the information. For many people, visual channels are the most effective and most frequently used. A nurse who observes that a patient looks pale and thin is using the visual communication channel, as is the person who reads a brochure about identifying skin cancer.

   ii. **auditory.** The second most commonly used communication channel is auditory, or hearing. This channel includes not only the words spoken but also how the words are spoken (for example, tone, pitch, etc.).

   iii. **kinesthetic.** This communication channel uses touch and other physiological responses to convey meaning. For example, a nurse touches the shoulder of a patient who is upset, to convey compassion. Or a nurse notices that a patient grimaces when she puts weight on her right leg. Touch can also be used to convey a number of emotions such as empathy, although it is important to remember that how people interpret touch varies significantly from culture to culture.

Nurse leaders are able to employ different channels as part of effective communication and leadership. Effective leaders are aware of the interactions of different channels as well as which channels may be more or less appropriate for different situations.

2. **Communication models.** According to Sullivan and Decker (1992), leaders use the following communication models to transmit information effectively from the sender to the receiver.

A. **Strategic choice model.** First described by Shelby (1988), this model
    suggests the following four strategic steps for helping leaders choose
    how they communicate messages to receivers:

    i.   identify communication goals (includes both information goals as
         well as goals of increasing the sender's credibility)
    ii. identify options (the possibilities available concerning style, pre-
         sentation, and channels to be used to convey the message)
    iii. assess probable response (leader analyzes the receivers' knowl-
         edge, personality, needs, attitudes, and cultural background that
         could affect how a message is received)
    iv. assess relative force (leader analyzes message effectiveness in meet-
         ing organizational goals, time required to deliver message, and
         whether the message quality is consistent with its significance)

B. **Cognitive management apparatus.** This model, also called the
    Targowski-Bowman model, is used to help understand the complexi-
    ties of communication within leadership or management settings.
    This model describes the different "links" the message moves through:

    i.   physical link. The actual physical connection between the receiver
         and the sender (for example, a telephone, face-to-face with voice,
         printed word)
    ii. systems link. The systems used to establish the physical link,
         including sender and receiver attitudes about these links
         a. For example, print media would be the systems link for a
             printed brochure, and it would include the attitudes people
             have about reliability, timeliness, or importance of print media
             and the reading level.
         b. A nurse leader who wanted to communicate to patients
             through a Web page, for example, would need to evaluate
             whether patients could access the Web, would be willing to do
             so, and believed that Web-based information was as reliable as
             a printed format.
    iii. audience link. This includes understanding the audience for the
         message and choosing the appropriate message for that audience.
         This link considers audience knowledge, perceptions, and size.
    iv. session link. Communication "time and space"—that is, whether
         a message is exchanged in real time (such as face-to-face, tele-
         phone, videoconference), or on a delay timeframe (e-mail, voice
         mail, written documents).
    v.   environmental link. The effect of surroundings on the communi-
         cation, for example in a public place vs. a private office or patient
         room.
    vi. functions/role link. The effect on messages of the organizational
         role and function of both sender and receiver. These roles can

include formal and informal status, and may also include economic or social hierarchies.

vii.   symbols link. Language and meaning and can include whether the sender and the receiver speak the same language (both literally and figuratively). Or it can include senders and receivers who speak the same language but who interpret nonverbal languages differently.

viii.   behavior link. Communicators evaluating observed behavior, especially the consistency (or inconsistency) between verbal and nonverbal messages. Not surprisingly, when the sender provides conflicting verbal and nonverbal messages, the receiver is more likely to believe the nonverbal message.

ix.   values link. The impact of an individual's personal and cultural values on how they receive and process information. For example, for one person with advanced cancer, "the best care" may be using every technological intervention available to prolong life. For another, "the best care" may consist of minimal technological or medical intervention and more emphasis on pain control and a dignified death.

x.   storage/retrieval link. Previous experiences of the sender and receiver and how they impact evaluation of messages. For example, a nurse leader who previously worked with a supervisor who withheld information as "punishment" may interpret a new supervisor's naturally quiet demeanor as critical or indicating dissatisfaction (Targowski & Bowman, 1988; Sullivan & Decker, 1992, pp. 120–121). Or, a staff member whose managers never called him into the office except for reprimands may be distracted for an entire shift if a new manager says, "Please stop by my office at the end of your shift," anticipating a negative interaction.

3. Communication modes. The main communication modes are verbal and nonverbal. In the most effective communication, verbal and nonverbal messages are compatible and not conflicting. Nonverbal messages are also strongly influenced by a person's culture and family, and cannot be interpreted in only one way.

A.   **Verbal communication** modes. The following are standard components of verbal communication.

i.   **word choice** consists of selecting appropriate words and arranging them in meaningful patterns. This includes using the language most familiar to the receiver.

a.   **accurate words** indicate the meaning clearly without confusion. Generally accurate words are concrete, specific, and do not have distracting connotations (emotional meanings).

For example, "sharp item" is not specific or clear—it could indicate a knife, a needle or, in some situations, a particularly good-looking outfit. Words such as "good" or "normal" often have emotional weight that goes beyond their official definition.

  b. **vocabulary** level of senders is also crucial. Using words that receivers do not comprehend means they will not understand the message. A nurse who has specialized vocabulary about medical procedures or leadership concepts needs to make sure that receivers understand this vocabulary. If they do not, it is the nurse leader's responsibility to use more common words until the message is comprehendible to receivers.

  ii. **tone** is the overall impression that words give. Tone is conveyed verbally by voice pitch (high or low), emphasis, and volume. Written tone is conveyed by word choice and sentence structure. Emoticons are symbols created from keyboard characters to convey nonverbal tone in e-mail messages in order to reduce misunderstandings and clarify communications. To indicate a joke or sarcasm, a wink is used: ;-) to indicate sadness, a frown can be used :- (Spoken and written tone can be formal or informal, friendly or distant, direct or indirect, enthusiastic or subdued. Tone has tremendous cultural variations—tone that is perceived as conversational in some countries is considered shouting in others.

  iii. speed or timing, or **pace.** This means how rapidly or slowly a person talks. In general, in the United States, rapid speaking conveys emotions such as excitement or frustration, while slower speech may be perceived as calming or boring.

  iv. written communication is the most conscious and controlled, followed by verbal communication. Nonverbal communication is the least conscious and controlled and therefore, most often clearly reveals a sender's true message and attitudes.

B.   **Nonverbal communication.** This consists of bodily, physical, and facial gestures that convey information. When the sender's verbal information and nonverbal information differ, the receiver may become confused or may choose to believe the nonverbal message (which is often perceived to be more genuine because of less conscious control). Nonverbal communications are very culture-specific. A nonverbal gesture in one culture or country may not mean the same thing as in another culture or country. The following are components of nonverbal communication.

  i. **body language**
    a. gestures: can be purposeful (such as waving hello) or inadvertent, such as fidgeting, waving hands, or crossing one's arms. These gestures can be interpreted differently according to situation, culture, and people involved. For example, a nurse supervisor crosses her arms across her chest while speaking.

Depending on the situation, this gesture could mean that the nurse is "closed" to communication. Or it could mean that the nurse is cold. In some cultures, this gesture is considered respectful while in others it is considered rude.

b. posture: how a person stands, sits, or moves. An erect posture can convey the message of assertiveness or confidence, while a slumped posture could mean fatigue, disinterest, or lack of confidence.

c. facial expressions: can include smiling, frowning, and whether the person maintains eye contact when speaking. Note that in the United States, making eye contact is considered essential to effective communication, but in many other cultures, direct eye contact between business associates or people of different ranks is seen as extremely rude.

ii. issues of **personal space.** This means the amount of space that people need to feel comfortable. Tremendous cultural differences exist in how much space people wish to maintain when talking to others, as well as appropriateness of touching another person. In the United States, touching someone in the workplace can be interpreted as sexual harassment. At the same time, touch is seen in some contexts as healing, calming, and therapeutic (Bovee & Thill, 2000).

iii. some body positions, postures, or gestures may be affected by physical conditions such as pain, neurological impairment, or orthopedic conditions.

iv. nurse leaders need to establish clear limits as to what body language and touching constitutes acceptable and unacceptable communication in the workplace. In health care, more than other work settings, physical touch is very common with patients, and therapeutic touch is an important tool in nursing care. Nurses may be so comfortable with the use of touch in their practice that they inadvertently offend another person when they use the same approach with someone who is not a patient.

4. Communication occurs in a variety of settings. Nurse leaders are aware of the complexity not only of the factors mentioned earlier, but also the impact of different communication settings in the workplace.

A. Communicating with people inside the organization

i. organizational roles. A person's role in an organization strongly affects how that person sends and receives information. These roles are usually categorized according to the organization's levels or hierarchies.

ii. hierarchies

a. **Upward communication** with superiors. Much upward communication consists of reporting information to facilitate problem-solving and decision-making. Nurse leaders must communicate effectively to their superiors or supervisors by stating their needs clearly, explaining the reason for their requests, and indicating benefits of the requested action.

b. **Downward communication** with subordinates. According to Sullivan & Decker (1992), successful downward communication relies on the following strategies:

   (i) know what needs to be done, who should do it, and steps needed to complete it. All of this information should appear in any instruction given to subordinates.

   (ii) eliminate as much interference as possible, allowing subordinates to listen effectively. Such interference may include internal resistance or external distractions.

   (iii) give information clearly and concisely, using appropriate vocabulary and nonoffensive voice tone, making sure that all needed information is included

   (iv) actively solicit feedback to ensure that subordinates have accurately and completely received the message

   (v) follow up by answering questions and verifying that tasks are being performed according to the instructions given

c. **Lateral (or horizontal) communication** with peers/coworkers, people at the same hierarchical level. This can include people from the same or other departments, such as pharmacists, respiratory, physical and occupational therapists. Although people at the same level usually share common experience, knowledge, and goals, it cannot be assumed that communication is automatic. Particularly given the increasing diversity of most departments, lateral communication still requires attention to the basics of the communication process.

d. **Diagonal communication** with people at different hierarchical levels within the organization but no direct supervisor/subordinate relationship (Sullivan & Decker, 1992, 2001), such as nurse-to-physician communication. A nurse may be at a lower hierarchical level than an attending physician, but not supervised by her; the same nurse may be at a higher hierarchical level than an intern, but not supervising him.

iii. **formal** and **informal** communication paths within organizations. People in organizations communicate through:

   a. official (formal) paths that are clearly documented and spelled out. These include official reporting mechanisms such as memos, e-mails, reports, etc.

   b. unofficial (informal) paths. These are the numerous ways that information makes its way through the organization.

Such "grapevine" information may be more or less accurate, and it is a powerful force in every organization. These informal communication paths are often instrumental in the politics of an organization, particularly during times of change or uncertainty.

iv. **public communication** (to small, medium, and large groups). The size of the receiving group affects how the message is organized and delivered. Generally, the larger the group, the more difficult the task of ensuring that the message is transmitted and received appropriately.

B. Communicating with patients and families. Nurse leaders must often deal with difficult situations that involve patients and their families, and disagreements or complaints about delivery of care. According to Sullivan and Decker (2001), nurse leaders should keep the following in mind when dealing with patient or family issues:

  i. Patients are customers and should be communicated with honestly and treated with respect. Even if the communication involves dealing with a complaint or other unpleasant scenario, the customer should receive prompt and tactful assistance.

  ii. Nurse leaders need to find a balance between avoiding medical jargon that is too complex and using terms that are too simple and condescending. Using the sender-message-receiver-feedback model, and paying attention to both verbal and nonverbal feedback will help nurse leaders negotiate this communication challenge.

  iii. Provide angry or upset customers a private, neutral place for communicating their needs.

  iv. When possible, if customers are not native speakers and/or not fluent in English, try to provide interpreter service. Professional interpreters (including those for American Sign Language) should be used whenever possible. Unless it is an emergency, do not use family members, as the practice is a potential violation of patient privacy. Furthermore, family members may have their own agendas and may not provide a literal translation, instead coloring the translation the way they want it to be transmitted to the patient. Seek guidance from your organization's compliance officer to stay up-to-date about patient care and privacy regulations as they relate to communicating with patients and others in the health care setting.

  v. Learn about different cultures in order to be able to recognize communication issues that are culturally based. A number of books about cross-cultural communication are published yearly. They are targeted at business travelers but are applicable to nurse leaders as well. Culturally-sensitive responses greatly increase communication with patients and families.

5. Tools that assist communication. Nurse leaders should know how to use the following basic communication tools.

A.   Written communication

   i.   memos, letters. A memo is usually a one-page communication targeted within an organization. It is meant to be brief and focused, covering one topic. Traditionally, memos have been the communication medium that organizations use to distribute information throughout the organization. Letters are one or more page communications addressed to readers outside the organization. Letters can perform a variety of functions including transmitting health information, fund-raising, or public relations.

   ii. brochures, patient information. Much patient education information continues to be in print form such as brochures or patient information booklets. These formats are generally longer, use a variety of print and graphic devices, and allow readers to access more complex information. It is critical that written patient information is at an eighth grade level or below (the national average reading level is about fifth grade) and that any illustrations are culturally sensitive and not stereotypical in any way.

B.   Electronic communication. Traditionally, all communication was either verbal or on paper. Electronic personal media devices are now found virtually everywhere and in some cases have replaced paper. The most frequently used electronic media include:

   i.   e-mail. For some time e-mails were considered strictly informal communication with little professional use, but now many organizations use e-mail for all internal and much of their external communications. Key points that nurse leaders need to remember about e-mail:
   a.   it has appropriate and inappropriate uses: Leaders need to develop clear policies and staff needs to be trained on what an organization considers as acceptable and unacceptable e-mail usage.
   b.   e-mail is not a universal substitute for face-to-face or real-time contact between people, such as by telephone
   c.   e-mails are stored electronically
   d.   any e-mail correspondence is the property of the organization and not of the sender or receiver
   e.   e-mail can be subpoenaed by the court

   ii. voice mail. Voice mailboxes that hold phone messages and allow retrieval through any other phone system are valuable ways of enhancing communication in organizations. As with e-mail, an organization needs clear policies on voice mail use. It should provide guidance and training for staff so that they can use this tool to facilitate communication without inappropriate diversion of organizational resources by extensive use for personal benefit outside the job requirements.

   iii. web-based information. Web-based communication can include an intranet that is usually password-protected for members of the organization only, and an Internet Web site that can be accessed by anyone inside or outside the organization.
   a. information about the organization—intranet and Internet
   b. link to related sites—intranet and Internet
   c. human resources information, policy and procedure manuals, clinical reference sources—intranet
   d. online training and education opportunities to meet organizational requirements—intranet
   e. patient information—Internet

C. Information systems. Computerized information systems provide patient monitoring and patient care tasks, as well as communication of data within the institution. According to Costello-Nickitas (1997), these tools not only enhance the quality of nursing care, they also help keep leadership on the cutting edge of patient care. Computerized systems include:

   i. **nursing information systems,** which contain nursing and health data that can be collected, stored, processed, retrieved, and communicated. These systems include
   a. patient classification
   b. care planning and documentation
   c. quality improvement
   d. inventory
   e. discharge planning
   f. performance measurement
   g. point of care systems.

   ii. **hospital information systems,** which manage information from clinical and administrative services such as patient accounting, financial management, patient care, pharmacy, radiology, and laboratories

   iii. **decision support systems,** which help leaders make informed operating decisions based on predictive data. These systems can include:
   a. cost accounting
   b. case mix information and acuity measurements to guide staffing requirements
   c. department and organization-wide budget and forecasting
   d. marketing

   iv. **executive information systems,** which allow leaders to explore key indicators such as performance, cash flow, capital expenditures, patient acuity, staffing levels, and patient and staff satisfaction

REVIEW ACTIVITIES

Questions

1. The exchange of information or opinions is referred to as
   a. feedback
   b. sender
   c. information systems
   d. communication

2. Which of the following is an element of Laswell's communication process model?
   a. interference
   b. culture
   c. message
   d. hierarchy

3. A nurse who initiates a conversation with a patient becomes which part of the communication process?
   a. feedback
   b. receiver
   c. sender
   d. message

4. The new message that is generated by the receiver in response to the original message from the sender is called
   a. clarity
   b. nonverbal communication
   c. feedback
   d. interruption

5. Which of the following principles about effective communication is true?
   a. giving information is the same as communication
   b. communication requires inactivity
   c. the receiver is responsible for message clarity
   d. feedback is essential even if it is not positive

6. When a receiver is distracted and does not fully receive the sender's message, this is called
   a. inattention
   b. indirect communication
   c. interaction
   d. interference

7. Three types of communication channels are
    a. television, radio, and e-mail
    b. visual, auditory, and kinesthetic
    c. sender, message, and receiver
    d. external, internal, and interactive

8. This communication channel uses touch or other physiological responses to convey meaning.
    a. visual
    b. mass
    c. auditory
    d. kinesthetic

9. The model used to help leaders understand the complexities of communication in leadership settings is called the
    a. strategic choice model
    b. cognitive management apparatus
    c. nonverbal communication model
    d. the time and space link model

10. In the Targowski-Bowman model, the link that accounts for the effect of surroundings on communication is the
    a. environmental link
    b. functions/role link
    c. physical link
    d. systems link

11. According to the storage-retrieval link of the Targowski-Bowman model,
    a. deals with speakers who use verbal and nonverbal language differently
    b. an individual's personal and cultural values affect how they process information
    c. previous experiences of sender and receiver influence how they evaluate messages
    d. deals with whether communications are exchanged in real time or on a delay

12. The overall impression that words give is the definition of
    a. word choice
    b. tone
    c. gesture
    d. pace

13. Which of the following is true about nonverbal communication?
    a. it is more conscious and deliberate than verbal communication
    b. it includes vocabulary, pace, and tone

    c. it is the same across most cultures

    d. it includes the issue of personal space

14. A nurse supervisor's communication with her staff in an organization is called

    a. downward

    b. upward

    c. lateral

    d. diagonal

15. Which of the following is true about lateral communication?

    a. it only includes people from different departments, not from the same department

    b. it requires little effort since people at the same level seldom share common knowledge and experience

    c. it cannot be used in diverse environments

    d. it requires attention to the basics of the communication process

16. Which of the following is not an electronic communication tool?

    a. intranet/web page

    b. a brochure

    c. voice mail

    d. e-mail

17. An information system that manages information from clinical and administrative services such as accounting, pharmacy, laboratory, etc, is called a

    a. hospital information system

    b. decision support system

    c. nursing information system

    d. executive information system

18. An executive information system would

    a. collect, store, and process patient classification and discharge planning data

    b. allow data for operating decisions such as case mix and marketing

    c. provide data for indicators such as capital expenditures and staffing levels

    d. distribute information about salaries of all supervisors

Critical Thinking Questions

1. A nurse in the emergency department needs to talk to a patient whose husband was very angry the last time the nurse spoke to them both. What nonverbal communication strategies could be used to convey the message that the husband needs to stay in control of his emotions?

2. What is a "show of force" in a health care setting? How can a show of force be used by a nurse?

3. Choose four patient education sheets or brochures produced by four different information providers. Analyze each for its ability to communicate information clearly, effectively and in a culturally sensitive manner.

4. Describe a situation in which you were misunderstood when you were talking to someone and another when you were using e-mail. What caused the misunderstanding? How could you reduce the risk of misunderstandings in the future?

5. When nurses speak to physicians, is it upward, downward or lateral communication? Provide a rationale for your answer.

Discussion Questions

1. Think of a conversation you recently had and label its components. Who was the sender? Who was the receiver? What was the message? Was there any feedback?

2. How does feedback affect communication where you work? What are the most common types or examples of feedback that you observe? Do they seem effective?

3. Divide your class into groups of three or four. In each group, choose one or two types of nonverbal communication. For each type of nonverbal communication, discuss the predominant "rules" for this communication, based on your particular culture. For example, what is the amount of personal space that is appropriate for your culture? What do certain gestures mean or convey?

4. For an organization or workplace in your community, diagram upward, downward, lateral, and diagonal communication. How are these types of communication alike? How are they different?

5. In your workplace, which communication tools do you use most often? Which are the most effective, and why?

Works Cited

Bovee, C. L., & Thill, J. V. (2004). *Business communication today* (6th ed.). Upper Saddle River, NJ: Pearson Education.

Costello-Nickitas, D. (1997). *Quick reference to nursing leadership*. Albany, NY: Thomson Delmar Learning.

Laswell, H. D. (1948). The structure and function of communication in society. In L. Bryson (Ed.), *The communication of ideas*. NY: Harper & Row.

Lucas, S. E. (2004). *The art of public speaking* (8th ed). Boston: McGraw-Hill.

Ruthman, J. L. (2003). Personal and interdisciplinary communication. In P. Kelly-Heidenthal (Ed.), *Nursing leadership & management* (pp. 119–139). Clifton Park, NY: Thomson Delmar Learning.

Shelby, A. (1988). A macro theory of management communication. *Journal of Business Communication, 25*(2), 13–27.

Sullivan, E. J., & Decker, P. J. (1992). *Effective management in nursing*. (3rd ed.). Redwood City, CA: Addison-Wesley Publishing.

Sullivan, E. J., & Decker, P. J. (2001). *Effective leadership and management in nursing* (5th ed.). Upper Saddle River, NJ: Prentice Hall.

Targowski, A., & Bowman, J. (1988). The layer-based, pragmatic model of the communication process. *Journal of Business Communication, 25*(1), 5–24.

Additional Resources

Bione, R. T., & Buck, R. (2003). Emotional expressivity and trustworthiness: The role of nonverbal behavior in the evolution of cooperation. *Journal of Nonverbal Behavior, 27*(3), 163–183.

Castledine, G. (2002). Medical language must be clarified for patients. *British Journal of Nursing, 11*(16), 1106.

Elfenbein, H. A., & Ambady, N. (2003). Cultural similarity's consequences: A distance perspective on cross-cultural differences in emotion recognition. *Journal of Cross-Cultural Psychology, 34*(1), 92–110.

Gudyknust, W. B. (Ed.). (2003). Cross-cultural and intercultural communication. Thousand Oaks, CA: Sage.

Hendrickson, S. G. (2003). Beyond translation . . . cultural fit. *Western Journal of Nursing Research, 25*(5), 593–608.

Ledger, S. D. (2002). Professional issues: Reflections on communicating with non-English-speaking patients. *British Journal of Nursing, 11*(11), 773–780.

Lipson, J. G., Dibble, S. L., & Minarik, P. A. (Eds.). (1996). *Culture and nursing care: A pocket guide*. San Francisco: UCSF Nursing Press.

Milstead, J. A. (2004). Challenging five traditional leadership principles. *Policy, Politics, & Nursing Practice, 5*(1), 5–10.

Pan American Health Organization. (2001). *Building standard-based information systems*. PAHO.

Strachan, H. (2004). Nursing information Communication. *Research and Theory for Nursing Practice, 18*(1), 7–10.

Wilkinson, K. T. (2004). Language difference and communication policy in the information age. *Information Society, 20*(3), 217–230.

Web Sites

AT&T Language Line Services
http://www.usa.att.com/traveler/access_numbers/
view.jsp?group=language

Center for Nonverbal Studies: National Communication Association
http://www.natcom.org/ctronline/nonverb.htm

Communication in Nursing
http://www06.homepage.villanova.edu/elizabeth.bruderle/
1103/communication.htm

Humanistic Nursing Communication Theory
http://www.samuelmerritt.edu/depts/nursing/duldt/

Journal of Communication
http://joc.oupjournals.org

Intercultural Communication Institute
http://www.intercultural.org

Nursing Communication Work Group: The Ottawa Hospital
http://www.ottawahospital.on.ca/hp/dept/nursing/npp/
wg/wg06-index-e.asp

Nursing Electronic Discussion Groups
http://www.sf.edu/nursing/links/communic.html

Society of Medical Interpreters
http://www.sominet.org

Taking IT Global
http://www.takingitglobal.org/themes/diversity/home.html

CHAPTER

7

COMMUNICATION SKILLS

active listening

anger

assertive

barriers

blaming

clarifying

conceding

conflict

culture

delineate

empathy

feedback

gender

identify

inattention

interrupting

nonverbal affirmation

questioning

rephrasing

resolve

responding

stereotyping

stress

verbal affirmation

INTRODUCTION

Nurse leaders facilitate communication for patients, families, nursing staff, other nurse leaders, and members of the health care team. This chapter provides information about more advanced skills that nursing leaders need as well as barriers that effective communicators must avoid or overcome.

KEY POINTS

1. Basic communication skills. Nursing leaders must have the necessary communication skills to work effectively with patients, families, other nurses, and members of the health care team, including superiors and subordinates.

According to Ruthman (2003), the key communication skills all nursing leaders need are:

A. **Active listening.** Sometimes called "attending," active listening requires:

    i. paying close attention to the speaker
    ii. noting both verbal and nonverbal messages (especially when they differ)
    iii. maintaining eye contact
    iv. avoiding behaviors that distract the listener and the speaker

B. **Responding.** The listener acknowledges in some way that he or she has received the message. Responding can include actions such as:

    i. **nonverbal affirmation,** such as nodding the head to indicate that the message has been received
    ii. **verbal affirmation,** such as "Yes" or "I hear you"
    iii. **questioning** to clarify the message; for example, "So you mean that. . .?"
    iv. **rephrasing** or restating the key points of the message, to affirm that the message has been received accurately. For example, "What I'm hearing is that. . . ."
    v. Questioning and rephrasing are considered more complex responses than nonverbal and verbal affirmation. They require:
        a. unwavering attention to the speaker
        b. that the listener does not jump in and take over the conversation. The questioning and rephrasing are built solely on the speaker's words, not the listener's thoughts or suggestions.

C. **Clarifying.** This skill allows listeners to accurately process information that may be disorganized or otherwise not clear. To clarify, the listener also uses restating and questioning—but this time to clear up any information that is confusing or contradictory, for example.

    i. restating. A patient relates a negative experience with hospital staff. The telling takes a while and the patient tends to go on tangents. The nurse leader can clarify that he or she has heard the main points by saying, "This is a lot of information, and I want to make sure I got it all. I'm going to repeat what I've heard, and you tell me if I have correctly understood you. OK?"
    ii. questioning. As with responding, this skill also allows the listener to clarify information that may not be completely clear when the speaker tells it. For example, the nurse leader may say, "Let me make sure I understand. The first week after you filled the prescription, you took 80 mg of nadolol every day—that was for seven days. And yesterday you had nausea and did not take any nadolol."

iii.   not surprising, these skills take time to learn. Nurse leaders also need to practice these skills frequently for them to be most effective.

D.   Dealing with **conflict.** Effective communication skills are also essential in resolving conflict. According to Ruthman (2003), the following three steps are essential for effectively dealing with conflict.

   i.   **identify** problem. Conflict arises from differences in opinions or perspectives. These differences can be real or perceived.
   a.   The effective nurse leader's first step in dealing with conflict is to be able to identify that a problem exists.
   b.   For example, one staff nurse perceives that the family members visiting Mrs. Waxman are upsetting her (because she cries when they come and go); while another staff nurse perceives that the tears are caused by joy rather than by distress. The nurse supervisor sees the nurses discussing whether Mrs. Waxman should have visitors and understands this is a problem and source of conflict.

   ii.   **delineate.** The next step in the process is to delineate, or to understand the problem and use knowledge and reason to resolve it.
   a.   This involves observation and gathering data.
   b.   For example, in this case, the nurse leader's task would be to talk with both nurses, with Mrs. Waxman and perhaps her family members. What is Mrs. Waxman's usual temperament (does she usually cry when joyful or is crying a sign of distress)? Do her vital signs change during or after visits? How many family members are visiting every day, for how long and at what times? How does the nurse leader perceive Mrs. Waxman's status? How do family members perceive it?

   iii.   **resolve.** Based on the observation that a problem exists, plus gathering of information about the problem, the final step is to try to resolve the problem.
   a.   Effective nurse leaders should try to make this process as much of a win-win for everyone as possible.
   b.   For example, based on discussions with all parties involved, observation and recording of Mrs. Waxman's vital signs, and the number of people visiting every day, the nurse leader decides that although Mrs. Waxman is probably cheered by expressions of concern, when more than two visitors are present, her heart rate and blood pressure increase. The nurse leader resolves this problem by communicating with staff nurses, Mrs. Waxman, and Waxman family members that only two people should visit Mrs.Waxman at one time and that the visitors should stay only 5–8 minutes, and why. The nurse leader communicates with the nursing staff and provides tips

on ways to deal with Waxman family members who might object to this policy.

E. Principles for effective active listening. According to Sullivan and Decker (1992), active listening requires the listener to pay more attention to taking in the message than to preparing or forming a response (not an easy task for people who are taught to solve problems). Following are eight key principles of active listening.

i. minimize distractions. It is difficult to listen in the focused way that active listening requires, with distractions present. To listen well, find a place that is quiet and where the listener and speaker will not be interrupted.

ii. look directly at the other person. The listener makes eye contact to let the speaker know that the listener is paying attention. (Note that people from different cultures have different tolerances for direct or sustained eye contact.)

iii. pay attention to both verbal and nonverbal messages. Although the listener is focused on the speaker's words, the listener also needs to pay close attention to nonverbal signals as well, especially if verbal and nonverbal signals are contradictory or confusing.

iv. ask questions to clarify if needed. Active listening uses questions to affirm that the listener has correctly received the speaker's meaning.

v. use empathy. **Empathy** means putting yourself in another person's place. Active listeners try to gain understanding by seeing the situation through the speaker's eyes.

vi. get **feedback** about what you are hearing. As discussed in chapter 6, the receiver generates a new message in response to the sender's original message. Active listening constantly uses feedback (through questioning and clarifying) to make sure the information is communicated clearly and accurately.

vii. acknowledge the other person's message and feelings. Active listening is a very nonjudgmental activity. The listener also needs to let the speaker know that he or she appreciates that this type of communication can be scary or tiring to the speaker. For example, the active listener can say to an impatient and angry father, "Mr. Fernandez, I know it is hard for you to have to wait for your son to have stitches, but the doctors have been tied up with two critical patients. As soon as one is available, he will be in here."

viii. be patient; avoid finding instant solutions. For people who are trained to find solutions, active listening can be a significant challenge, as it asks the listener to listen and avoid finding solutions. Effective active listeners must train themselves to be patient and receptive and to wait for the speaker to communicate his or her thoughts and needs.

F. Advanced communication skills. Appropriately assertive behavior plus consistent active listening allow the nurse leader to practice advanced communication skills, which can be used in the most challenging communication settings. According to Ruthman (2003), these skills include:

    i. focusing—keeping communications on track by reiterating the key point or points, for example, by saying "So your main concern is. . . ."

    ii. providing information to people that they did not previously have. For example, a family is concerned about their 70-year-old mother's "erratic" behavior after being hospitalized for a urinary tract infection. The nurse leader explains to them that infection and dehydration can cause this behavior and that their mother is not necessarily developing dementia.

    iii. reassuring—helping restore confidence or decreasing fear; for example, reassuring a patient that he or she will feel significantly better in about 12 hours, after the effects of procedural sedation have worn off.

    iv. using appropriate humor—if used correctly, humor can decrease tension and help a patient or family member regain perspective. Note that humor is generally not cross-cultural and not all people appreciate it in all settings. Making fun of oneself is often the most successful approach to humor. Take your lead from the people around you.

    v. expressing acceptance or appreciation—letting patients or family know that a behavior (such as crying) is OK, or simply saying "thank you."

    vi. asking questions to expand the listener's understanding. For example, the nurse leader may say, "Mrs. DiNoia, can you tell me what you remember about your visit to Dr. Appleton's office last week?"

G. Being appropriately **assertive** in communicating with others. Assertiveness in communication means the ability to stand up for one's rights and needs without violating the rights of others. According to Smith (1975), the following behaviors are appropriate to professionally assertive communication:

    i. do not apologize unless you are clearly at fault, or you know who is at fault and you are taking responsibility for what happened

    ii. avoid reactions such as tantrums, revenge, sarcasm, and threats, which increase listeners' defensiveness and decrease speaker's ability to communicate effectively

    iii. make sure that nonverbal and verbal messages are consistent

    iv. avoid a knee-jerk reaction to negative responses or criticism from patients, staff, or family

    v. use "I" statements to convey feelings, and be honest about feelings, needs, or ideas

    vi. acknowledge faults but do not overly apologize for them

2. Communication **barriers.** According to Ruthman (2003), there are a number of obstacles to effective communication. The nurse leader who is aware of and can identify the presence of these barriers is more able to avoid or compensate for them.

    A. **Culture.** Nursing staffs and patient populations are increasingly diverse, coming from different parts of the world, following different religious observances, varying practices and rituals, avoiding different taboos, and eating or avoiding certain types of food. Poole, Davidhizar, and Giger (1995) note that the following concepts are present in all cultures:

        i. communication. Language or dialect, rules about what is appropriate conversational volume, words that can be said in public, and whether people can touch when they communicate

        ii. space. The socially appropriate space between people (how much space is needed while speaking face to face or eating) or how much space is acceptable with different types of relationships (married or intimate, kin, friend, nurse)

        iii. social organization. Is the family or the individual the primary unit of social organization? For example, in determining treatment for a patient, does the culture focus on using all means to save the person, or does the culture focus on the total impact on the person's extended family?

        iv. time. Does the culture look more toward the past, the present, or the future? Different cultures use time differently, as well. Some cultures value timeliness and punctuality, while other cultures value fluidity and flexibility, with "clock time" a distant second or third in importance.

        v. environmental control. Does the culture perceive control as being inside the person (for example, the concept of individualism or free will) or does the culture perceive control as existing outside the person (in the hands of a deity or a power such as destiny or fate)?

        vi. biological variations. This recognizes that different ethnic and cultural groups have inherited varied tendencies; for example, susceptibility or resistance to certain diseases; for example, African Americans are more likely to have high blood pressure than any other group.

    B. Emotions. These are frequently barriers to communication, as they prevent people from listening and speaking effectively. According to Ruthman (2003)

     i. **anger** is a strong feeling of displeasure that results from a situation which prevents a person from getting what is wanted. Anger maybe justified but it is also disruptive and, if not controlled, can be destructive.

    ii. other emotion-based responses include:

       a. **blaming,** or finding fault with another's actions; blaming usually indicates a lack of respect for others' feelings

       b. placating, or **conceding** means that the placater does not stand up for his or her rights and essentially says, "I'm always wrong, you're right."

C. **Gender.** Although controversy continues about how alike and different men and women actually are, most agree that men and women tend to communicate differently. According to Sullivan and Decker (2001), the differences in male and female communication include:

     i. speaking style (men tend to speak more, longer and faster)

    ii. spoken message content (females describe more, clarify more, and use questions)

   iii. managing conflict (men tend to disagree more, while women tend to seek cooperation)

   iv. relating to others (women respond more to subordinates, while men respond more to superiors)

    v. Blanchard and Sargent (1986) argue that the best leaders are "androgynous"—able to combine the best traits of female and male communication styles

D. **Conflict.** Another barrier to effective communications is conflict. According to Ruthman (2003), conflict arises when a person's beliefs or ideas are opposed. Conflict can occur between persons, persons and organizations, and among organizations. In general, when conflict occurs, people

     i. tend to stop communicating effectively (or not at all)

    ii. use ineffective conflict resolution or management techniques (see Chapter 10, Conflict Resolution Skills, for more information)

E. Other communication barriers.

     i. **stress,** a state of tension that gets in the way of reasoning. People under stress do not listen well and often may not send clear messages.

    ii. **stereotyping,** an unfair categorizing of someone based on his or her cultural, racial, or gender traits; for example, "You just can't reason with women; they're too emotional."

   iii. **interrupting** rather than listening occurs when the listener gives feedback before the speaker has finished delivering the message. A person may interrupt because he or she is eager to speak, but in most contexts, interrupting does not lead to effective communication.

  iv. not paying attention, or **inattention**, means that the listener may miss key parts of the message. Inattention may also send the message to the speaker that his or her message is not important or worthy of the listener's time.

3. Future trends affecting communication.

  A. Diversity. As discussed earlier, different assumptions and influences can be barriers to communication when the speaker or listener is not aware that these differences exist. As the workplace and patient population becomes increasingly diverse, nurse leaders will need to be aware of the following trends.

  i. cultural diversity. Even in small communities, there may be dozens of different ethnic and cultural communities, each with its own practices about communication, food, medical practices, hygiene, etc. Demographic indicators show that this will become even more of a factor in coming years.

  ii. religious diversity. Different religious practices affect people's willingness to undergo treatment, how they view different parts of the body, their perspective on different medications (pharmaceutical vs. herbal, for example) as well as how much (if any) treatment they are willing to undergo.

  iii. familial diversity. The "traditional" nuclear family of one male parent, one female parent (married to each other), and two children is no longer the norm. According to Carroll (2004), families today may consist of unmarried opposite sex partners, an array of closely-related or loosely knit kin, neighbors, same-sex partners, intergenerational groups, multicultural or multiracial groups.

  B. Aging population. As people grow older, they have more illnesses, and may be more limited in their ability to hear and speak. These changes affect their ability to communicate effectively. Nurse leaders need to be aware of this trend and adapt their communication skills accordingly.

  C. Ongoing and rapid changes in technology. As discussed in Chapter 6, the trend is toward electronic communication, including e-mail, voice mail, cell phones, and handheld devices, all of which can make communication more and less effective. Further, people with less education, those in rural areas, and people with low incomes have less access to technology-assisted communication—an important factor to consider when working with staff members at different levels in an organization and with patients of various backgrounds.

Nurse leaders need to be aware of available tools, while remembering that no tool replaces the key skills of active listening, giving and receiving feedback, and being aware of and working around barriers that can impede effective communication.

REVIEW ACTIVITIES

Questions

1. Which of the following is a component of active listening?
   a. paying close attention to the speaker
   b. providing advice to help the speaker solve his or her problem
   c. inviting others to join the conversation to clarify issues
   d. focusing on the words spoken

2. An example of rephrasing would be
   a. "Yes, I hear you."
   b. "So when you say 'a lot' you mean twice a day?"
   c. "What I hear you say is. . . ."
   d. "I don't understand you."

3. The active listening skill of clarifying allows the listener to
   a. tell the speaker what to do
   b. restate what the speaker previously said
   c. accurately process information that maybe disorganized or confusing
   d. interrupt the speaker

4. The three essential steps for dealing with conflict are
   a. identify, understand, and resolve the problem
   b. listen actively, provide solution, and suppress any anger
   c. restate, question, and clarify the speaker's statement
   d. identify, negotiate, and rephrase the listener's response

5. Putting yourself in another person's place is called
   a. delineation
   b. active listening
   c. feedback
   d. empathy

6. The advanced communication skill of keeping a conversation on track is also known as
   a. rephrasing
   b. focusing

    c. humor

    d. reassuring

7. Assertive behavior is characterized by:

    a. apologizing frequently

    b. sarcasm

    c. standing up for one's rights

    d. blaming others

8. Communication barriers can consist of:

    a. cultural, emotional, or gender issues

    b. overuse of "I" statements

    c. respecting and following other people's cultural preferences

    d. paying attention to what people say

9. The communication barrier that occurs when a person is categorized according to his or her gender, cultural, or racial traits is called:

    a. blaming

    b. conflict

    c. inattention

    d. stereotyping

Critical Thinking Questions

1. A patient's daughter comes to the nurse's station and asks to speak to the nurse in charge. She is upset and angry because her mother is very upset about her new diagnosis of cancer, yet the family of the patient sharing the room is boisterous and laughing. How should a nurse leader handle this situation?

2. Lawyers who evaluate malpractice cases state that patients often come to them because they feel the hospital or health care provider is trying to hide something when there is a complication or undesirable outcome. How should a nurse leader handle a situation in which a patient develops a rash after she receives the wrong drug? What should be done if the patient falls because of a drop in blood pressure related to a medication error?

3. When patients and families are faced with a sudden hospitalization, tempers often flare and people are much more sensitive to the length of time they must wait. Families may also be troubled by standard rules in a hospital, such as visiting hours and policies. How can the nurse leader mitigate these situations and use communication skills to keep these situations under control?

Discussion Questions

1. In an organization where you work (or have worked), think of someone who practices active listening. What does that person do to show that he or she is listening? What impact does the listening have on people who are being listened to?

2. For an organization that you know well, what are the primary communication barriers? How might these barriers be reduced or overcome?

Works Cited

Blanchard, K. H., & Sargent, A. G. (1986). The one-minute manager is an androgynous manager. *Nursing Management, 17*(5), 44–45.

Carroll, P. (2004). *Community health nursing: A practical guide.* Clifton Park, NY: Thomson Delmar Learning.

Poole, V. L., Davidhizar, R. E., & Giger, J. N. (1995). Delegating to a transcultural team. *Nursing Management, 26*(8), 33–34.

Ruthman, J. L. (2003). Personal and interdisciplinary communication. In P. Kelly-Heidenthal (Ed.), *Nursing leadership & management* (pp. 119–139). Clifton Park, NJ: Thomson Delmar Learning.

Smith, M. (1975). *When I say no, I feel guilty.* New York: Bantam.

Sullivan, E. J., & Decker, P. J. (1992). *Effective management in nursing* (3rd ed.). Redwood City, CA: Addison-Wesley Publishing.

Sullivan, E. J., & Decker, P. J. (2001). *Effective leadership and management in nursing* (5th ed.). Upper Saddle River, N.J.: Prentice Hall.

Additional Resources

Bush, K. (2001). Do you really listen to patients? *RN, 64*(3), 35–37.

Dawes, B. Communicating nursing care and crossing language barriers. *AORN Journal,* May 2001. Retrieved 7/2/04 from http://www.findarticles.com/p/articles/mi_m0FSL/is_5_73/ai_74571575

Gray, J. (1992). *Men are from Mars, women are from Venus.* New York: HarperCollins.

Gudyknust, W. B. (Ed.). (2003). *Cross-cultural and intercultural communication.* Thousand Oaks, CA: Sage.

Klagsbrun, J. (2001). Listening and focusing: Holistic health care tools for nurses. *Nursing Clinics of North America, 36*(1), 115–129.

Ledger, S. D. (2002). Professional issues: Reflections on communicating with non-English-speaking patients. *British Journal of Nursing, 11*(11), 773–780.

Lipson, J. G., Dibble, S. L., & Minarik, P. A. (Eds.). (1996). *Culture and nursing care: A pocket guide*. San Francisco: UCSF Nursing Press.

Michaels, C. L. (2002). Circle communication: An old form of communication useful for 21st century leadership. *Nursing Administration Quarterly, 26*(5), 1–10.

Morrison, T., Conway, W. A., & Borden, G. A. (1995). *Kiss, bow, or shake hands: How to do business in 60 countries*. 1994 Adams Media Corporation Avon, MA.

Tannen, D. (2001). *You just don't understand me: Men and women in conversation*. New York: Quill.

Tannen, D.(1995). *Gender and discourse*. Oxford: Oxford University Press.

Tate, D. M. (2003). Cultural awareness: Bridging the gap between caregivers and Hispanic patients. *Journal of Continuing Education in Nursing, 34*(5), 213–217.

Web Sites

Active Listening Skills Taft College, CA
    http://www.taft.cc.ca.us/lrc/class/assignments/actlisten.html

Communication Boosters: Center for American Nurses
    http://www.nursingworld.org/can/tools/boosters.htm

The Communications Doctor
    http://www.communicationsdoctor.com/articles.html

Express Healthcare Management: Importance of Communication
    http://www.expresshealthcaremgmt.com/20040131/conversation02.shtml

Leadership and Communication
    http://www.nwlink.com/~donclark/leader/leadcom.html

Leadership, Communication and Change
    http://www.work911.com/articles/comchan.htm

Principles for Leadership Communication
    http://was4.hewitt.com/hewitt/resource/articleindex/talent/principles.htm

CHAPTER

8

DECISION-MAKING AND TIME-MANAGEMENT TOOLS

analyze

benefits

certainty

consensus

consequences

critical thinking

decision-making

decision tree

Delphi group

Gantt chart

goal

matrix

maximax approach

maximin approach

nominal group

perspective

probability

Program Evaluation and Review Technique (PERT) flowchart

risk

risk averting approach

stakeholders

uncertainty

INTRODUCTION

All leaders must make decisions and the most effective leaders have a strategic plan for gathering information, evaluating information, and deciding a course of action, based on critical thinking. Time management is a critical skill that requires a constant series of effective decisions. Not surprisingly, leaders who think and decide effectively also tend to use their time more effectively.

KEY POINTS
Decision-Making Skills

1. Definition

    A.   **Decision-making** is the process of establishing criteria by which a nurse leader can develop and select a course of action from a group of alternatives.

        i. decisions may or may not be the result of "problems"
       ii. decision-making is considered a critical thinking process, just like problem solving

    B.   Characteristics of decision-making

        i. not a linear or totally logical process; may involve intuition as well
       ii. is often the result of many incremental steps rather than one large step
      iii. smaller choices may be impacted by many factors other than rationality and analytical thought (Sullivan & Decker, 1992; Little-Stoetzel, 2003)

    C.   Characteristics of successful decision makers

        i. learn to emphasize the tools and techniques that help make decision-making effective and efficient
       ii. minimize the techniques or events that can sidetrack the critical thinking/decision-making process
      iii. ability to engage in **critical thinking** is the foundation for decision-making and problem solving success

    D.   Effective critical thinkers

        i. constantly generate new ideas and alternatives
       ii. do not rely on "we've always done it this way"
      iii. are able to step back from issue and **analyze** (separate and examine) its components. They often ask:
          a. What are the underlying assumptions of this point of view?
          b. Where does the evidence come from and how is it being interpreted?
          c. How does the logic or argument hold together?
       iv. can discern the quality of information that underlies ideas—whether it is precise, accurate, relevant, consistent, logical, complete, and unbiased
       v. are able to assume another person's **perspective** or point of view in order to see all sides of an issue (Sullivan & Decker, 1992)

2. Successful decision-making tends to follow a series of strategic steps, including:

  A.   Identify the need for a decision. This step should consider:

   i.   what needs to be determined
   ii.   why a decision is needed
   iii.   all the information available
   iv.   try to state issues in broader terms rather than narrower terms
   v.   for example, a visiting policy may allow only one family member to be with a patient at a time. However, the patient is 15 years old and his single mother is with his 10-year-old brother because she did not have anyone else to stay with the younger boy.

  B.   Determine the desired **goal** or outcome. The goal should be:

   i.   clear and specific
   ii.   stated in a sentence or two
   iii.   in the above example, the goal or outcome is to decide if making an exception to hospital policy is in this patient's best interest. It is also reasonable to determine if the hospital's goals concerning patient care and privacy can be met if an exception to the policy is allowed.

  C.   Identify any other actions that exist. For each alternative action, identify:

   i.   its possible **consequences** (negative impacts)
   ii.   its possible **benefits** (positive impacts)
   iii.   this step may also include evaluating the quality of evidence and existing arguments for or against an alternative action
   iv.   in this example, the benefit of allowing the second visitor is additional support for the patient since he and his brother are close, and not having a 10-year-old by himself in a waiting area. Possible consequences could be loss of privacy and inconsistency with other patients' visitors.

  D.   Decide which action to implement, based on each action's benefits and consequences.

   i.   For multiple choices or complex alternatives, it may be helpful to use a rating or ranking system to help prioritize benefits and consequences.
   ii.   In the above example, depending on liability and other issues, the nursing staff may rank issues of consistency with all visitors and privacy for the other patient in the room higher. Or the staff may decide that patient comfort and keeping the family together rank higher.

E. Evaluate the action by asking these questions:

    i. was the goal achieved completely?

    ii. was the goal achieved partially?

    iii. was the goal not achieved at all? (Little-Stoetzel, 2003).

    iv. for this example, if the decision was to allow the second visitor, did having a second visitor present make the patient less anxious? Did it not seem to make a difference either way? Or did the additional family member actually make the patient more anxious?

    v. effective decision makers always attempt to see and think about the complex interactions that occur in decision-making as well as the ripple effect; that is, the impact of the decision beyond the immediate issue and develop strategies that ensure the most beneficial outcomes for all parties affected by the decision.

3. Decision-making may change under differing conditions. Possibilities include:

A. Under conditions of **certainty**

    i. alternatives and existing conditions are well known

    ii. decision can be made with full knowledge of what the outcome will be

    iii. conditions of certainty are rare in health care but they do exist; for example, evidence-based knowledge about the use of standard precautions to reduce transmission of infectious diseases

B. Under conditions of **risk**

    i. alternatives and conditions are not very well known

    ii. decision outcome can only be expressed as **probability** (likelihood) rather than certainty. The key to this analysis is, understanding different levels of probability:

        a. objective probability. likelihood that an event will or will not occur based on facts and reliable information

        b. subjective probability. likelihood that an event will or will not occur based on a leader's personal judgment and beliefs

        c. for example, when choosing vendor services, objective probability that the vendor will perform effectively can be established through researching the vendor's track record, talking with past and current customers, and evaluating the vendor's responsiveness to questions. Subjective probability would be based on a supervisor's friendship with, loyalty to, or previous positive experiences with a vendor's sales representative.

C. Under conditions of **uncertainty**

    i. alternatives and conditions are complex and variable; the person making the decision may not even be aware of all the possibilities, or the decision-making may be occurring in a rapidly changing environment

ii. decision outcome cannot be expressed even as a probability (Sullivan & Decker, 2001)

iii. for example, when anthrax was used as a bioweapon in 2001, decisions about treatment and protection of the public were made under conditions of uncertainty with no precedent and only theoretical models to guide public health officials

4. According to Sullivan and Decker (1992), there are three approaches for dealing with conditions of uncertainty—the typical condition for many health care settings:

A. **Maximax approach** (most optimistic)

   i. Select the alternative with the best possible outcome for all alternatives

   ii. For example, to ensure expert operating room staffing for a complex procedure for which technology is rapidly changing, continue to recruit and retain the best possible staff, even though the procedure may change in the future

B. **Maximin approach** (most pessimistic)

   i. Choose the worst possible outcome for each possible alternative

   ii. Then choose the least objectionable worst outcome

   iii. Using this approach, the nurse leader might decide that the complex procedure will become obsolete and stop providing any staff support or training for the procedure

C. **Risk averting approach**

   i. Select the alternative that has the fewest variables among its possible outcomes

   ii. This approach is considered highly effective

   iii. For example, in this case, the nurse leader might decide to recruit a small, experimental staff at first, who could train others in the procedure (if demand for the procedure continued or grew) or these staff members could move into other positions (if demand for the procedure decreased)

5. How novices and experts make decisions differently. According to Benner (1984)

A. Effective decision makers

   i. understand the link between information, thinking, and good decisions

    ii. understand that decisions can change as information or situations change

    iii. anticipate questions, opposition, alternatives, and outcomes

    iv. use their experience and learning as a foundation for good decision-making

    v. are creative

B.   The link between decision-making and patient care

    i. nurses review care selections available, choose the best option, and implement that option for patients

    ii. decision-making (which may or may not involve an immediate "problem") is a major part of a nurse's work in patient care

    iii. nurses are also key to helping patients take a more active role in making decisions about their own health. Patients involved in the decision process are more likely to follow treatment plans, leading to better outcomes.

C.   Decision-making and leadership/management issues

    i. leaders and managers often face complex decision-making scenarios (many possible alternatives/actions and a variety of benefits or consequences)

    ii. leaders often use a **matrix,** which lists actions, alternatives, benefits, and consequences in a table or graphic form, for easy comparison

    iii. in some cases, scores are assigned to each action and consequences, to help prioritize or weigh options

    iv. leaders often use visual decision-making tools, such as:

        a. **Program Evaluation and Review Technique (PERT) flow-charts,** which show the amount of time taken and the sequence of events needed to complete the project

        b. **decision trees,** which show all the outcomes and benefits of a particular decision

        c. **Gantt charts,** which graphically illustrate a project from start to finish, including time intervals for interim steps (Little-Stoetzel, 2003).

6. Decision-making within groups

A.   Depending on the decision and its consequences, it may be appropriate for a nurse leader to make decisions with a group rather than alone. Group decisions must include the **stakeholders,** the people who will be affected by the decision.

    i. Advantages of group decision-making: more people involved, more input and feedback, more stakeholders who can "buy in" to decision and outcome and support the group's decision

ii. Disadvantages of group decision-making: time consuming, can be poor use of time if decision process is not well-managed; in some cases it can lead to increased conflict and sabotage of the group's decision

B.   Methods of group decision-making

    i. **consensus** building
       a. all group members can live with and fully support the decision
       b. consensus does not mean that everyone agrees, it just means that they can live with it
       c. advantages include greater support for decisions made
       d. disadvantages include time needed for decisions and that people wanting to block a decision can use consensus to delay decisions

    ii. **nominal group** technique
       a. primarily nonverbal technique in which group members write out their ideas
       b. these ideas and their pros and cons are presented on a flip board or chart
       c. group discusses ideas and then puts them to a private vote; the highest rating wins

    iii. **Delphi group** technique
       a. group members receive questionnaire (no face-to-face meeting)
       b. results are summarized and redistributed
       c. process of questionnaire followed by summary continues until the group reaches consensus
       d. this technique allows large numbers of people to be involved and reduces conflict that can arise with face-to-face meetings, but it can take much longer

C.   Groupthink

    i. type of decision-making that depends on getting everyone to agree totally
    ii. discourages disagreement and creative problem solving
    iii. symptoms of groupthink include a group feeling that
       a. the group is always right
       b. outsiders are stereotypically wrong
       c. any outside evidence that refutes the group's stand can and should be dismissed regardless of its merit

D.   Effective group decision-making depends on

    i. all group members having the freedom to think for themselves
    ii. all group members being able to state their opinions and ideas freely
    iii. groups having time to collect data and reflect on it (Little-Stoetzel, 2003)

E.   Obstacles to effective decision making include:

i.   not exploring all information available

ii.   taking into account or presenting only biased information

iii.   seeking to avoid change or conflict

iv.   using new decisions to justify previous decisions made (especially if experience shows that the previous decisions were inadequate or incorrect)

v.   failing to accurately represent the consequences of preferred actions or benefits of alternative actions (Sullivan & Decker, 1992)

7. Decisions and technology

A.   Technology can help sort, organize, track, and analyze data:

i.   decision-making grids in Excel or Word

ii.   databases to store multiple and complex data sets

iii.   software that allows quick and easy manipulation of data:
a.   decision trees
b.   Gantt charts
c.   project management software

B.   However, technology cannot perform critical thinking tasks and that is up to the nurse leader.

KEY TERMS: TIME MANAGEMENT

brainstorming

critical outcomes

intermediate outcomes

nonurgent outcomes

Pareto principle

personal strategies

time management

KEY POINTS
Time-Management Skills

1. Definition

A.   **Time management** skills are those actions that help nurses use their time most effectively and productively

i.   achieving more with the time that is available

    ii. requires the following actions:
      a. prioritizing tasks
      b. analyzing how time is being used
      c. assessing distractions that detract from effective time use

B. Time management also includes the larger concepts of

    i. clarifying vision
    ii. identifying goals (short-range and long-range)
    iii. organizing and implementing tasks to reach the targeted vision

C. A key concept of time management is the **Pareto principle:**

    i. 20% of focused efforts results in 80% of outcomes
    ii. 80% of unfocused efforts results in 20% of outcomes
    iii. the key is to focus effort on the activities that will get the maximum results

D. An effective time-management strategy consists of:

    i. using results rather than tasks as more accurate way to measure effectiveness of time use
    ii. breaking long-term goals into short-term, achievable outcomes
    iii. the ability to change outcomes or goals when previous goal becomes unrealistic

E. How nurses actually use their time. According to Maloney (2003), studies have shown that:

    i. Acute care nurses spend 30–35% of their time on direct care, 25% on charting and reporting, and the remainder (slightly less than half) of their time on admission and discharge procedures, communication, and miscellaneous actions (Upenieks, 1998)
    ii. RNs spend around 30% of time on direct care, around 40% on indirect care, 15% on unit maintenance activities, and 15% on other activities not related to patient care or unit maintenance (Urden & Roode, 1997)
    iii. Nurses' recall of how time is spent is generally not accurate; the most accurate way to track actual time usage is through an activity log or with people monitoring and tracking tasks and behaviors

2. Strategies for more effective use of time include:

A. Use a "big picture" perspective

    i. understand that nurses do not work in isolation: they work with other nurses, technicians, and other heath professionals and support staff

    ii. what nurses do is also impacted by what is happening on the unit, outside the unit, and in the organization

    iii. understanding the dynamics of the larger situation allows nurses to be more flexible and make decisions that fit more than just a narrow range of needs

B. Use **brainstorming** to see total tasks and to break them into reasonable, smaller goals

    i. this technique allows the nurse leader to use creativity in time management and decision-making

    ii. brainstorming, facilitated properly, encourages thinking outside the box and may reveal solutions that were not previously obvious

C. Decide on outcomes. These need to be:

    i. optimal. best possible results given the resources available

    ii. reasonable. the best that can be expected if optimal results are not available due to crises, unusual circumstances, etc

D. Prioritize outcomes in order of importance. According to Hansten and Washburn (1998), once nurse leaders choose outcomes, they must assign tasks according to importance:

    i. **critical:** life threatening or potentially life threatening, such as a patient who is in cardiac or respiratory arrest, respiratory or advanced cardiac failure, or related situations that affect airway, breathing and circulation, such as life-threatening hemorrhage or other intravascular fluid loss

    ii. **intermediate:** usually activities essential for patient safety, including availability of lifesaving medications and equipment, as well as actions that protect patients from infection and injury

    iii. **nonurgent:** activities needed to complete the plan of care to relieve symptoms or lead to healing and prevent complications, such as positioning and patient teaching

E. According to Costello-Nickitas (1997), there are six key steps that allow nurses to prioritize their work and time to accomplish "first things first":

    i. deal with interruptions openly and directly

       a. refuse to get involved with interruptions that detract from important tasks

       b. communicate your philosophy clearly to others (for example, "I enjoy talking with you but I have a report to finish by mid-afternoon.")

    ii. improve efficiency of telephone communications

       a. use voice mail or other methods to screen calls

       b. set aside blocks of time to return calls

       iii. keep meetings on track
          a. send agenda before meeting
          b. keep meeting on track with agendas; place issues that arise from the meeting on the next meeting's agenda
          c. start and stop on time
       iv. reduce the paper trail
          a. use the "one touch" system for all papers—touch them only once, then either decide, delegate, or discard
          b. keep piles of paper off desk
          c. encourage others to reduce their paper load to you; for example, do you need to receive copies of minutes for every meeting? Do you need to receive copies of standard correspondence?
       v. block out time for important activities
          a. for special projects set a time and date to work on them; gather any needed material beforehand
          b. make workspace a "do not disturb" area for a set time; during this time, avoid talking with visitors, responding to e-mails, or answering the phone
       vi. reduce clutter
          a. avoid letting papers and other items pile up in the work area
          b. discard unnecessary items
          c. file remaining items according to their importance or priority
          d. label files clearly so that materials are easy to find

F. Once the nurse leader commits to a time management strategy, it is essential to stay focused on that goal. Tools for staying focused include:

       i. allowing intuition to become a part of thinking, in addition to analysis
       ii. using brainstorming or other ways to generate ideas about breaking down larger goals into smaller, more manageable tasks
       iii. creating a personal mission statement that provides overall direction and reflects commitment to patients and team members (Costello-Nickitas, 1997)
       iv. seeking out a professional mentor who has these skills and who can provide constructive, confidential feedback

3. Workplace strategies for applying time management skills to delivery of care

A. Determine how long tasks or activities actually take

       i. may combine estimates and observation
       ii. most people tend to underestimate time spent on tasks
       iii. accurate estimates allow for more realistic planning

B. Create supportive environment for time management and best patient care, including:

  i. locating supplies or other materials so that the staff can access them easily and without repetitive or additional effort; for example, preassembled kits for procedures significantly reduce time spent on collecting needed items
  ii. establishing protocols, checklists, etc. to help nurses or other staff plan and organize a task
  iii. helping the staff distinguish between essential and nonessential tasks, or tasks to be performed by different levels of personnel

C. Create shift summaries to document what actually occurs on a shift. These reports can be gathered from conversations, taped reports, and through making patient rounds.

  i. advantages: allows clarification and communication about patient status, planning, and nurses' questions
  ii. disadvantages: takes time, and discussions can be sidetracked onto other nonpatient issues
  iii. based on this information, nurse leaders can produce shift action plans that address outcomes, set priorities, and specify essential care actions based on these outcomes and priorities

D. Evaluate outcome achievement

  i. at the end of the shift, the nurse leader reexamines the shift action plan and determines if goals were accomplished
  ii. common reasons that goals are not accomplished include procrastination, poor delegation, indecisiveness, poor time management (Maloney, 2003) as well as unpredictable shifts in workload, such as admissions and patient crises

4. Personal strategies for increasing time management and productivity

A. Create time

  i. learn to say "no" to others
  ii. eliminate work that does not help achieve outcomes
  iii. delegate when feasible and appropriate

B. Use downtime effectively

  i. try to avoid getting stuck waiting, by calling ahead to verify appointments, and by arriving not more than five minutes early for appointments
  ii. if forced to wait, have materials available to work on, read; or return phone calls/leave messages, if appropriate

      iii. use downtime moments for "mental breaks," deep breathing, or other stress reduction or reenergizing techniques

      iv. on the clinical unit, use downtime for restocking, cleaning up, organizing unit workspaces and reading professional journals or reviewing policies and procedures

C. Control or minimize distractions

      i. use techniques to discourage casual visitors, such as meeting visitors at the door, standing in front of your desk, making the office less inviting, or removing visitor's chair from the area

      ii. have certain "closed door" times in the office, signaling no interruptions with a note or sign on the door

      iii. use answering machine or voice mail to limit phone accessibility; be sure to set blocks of time aside to return phone calls

      iv. encourage others to be more independent and to reduce interruptions when they ask for assistance

D. Use opportunities to increase or practice skills

      i. try to find ways to do "old" tasks in new, more efficient ways

      ii. take advantage of formal and informal learning opportunities

      iii. develop computer skills that allow you to perform tasks more easily and efficiently

E. Learn and use paper and electronic tools for scheduling and managing time

      i. daily and monthly calendars
         a. yearly calendars for long-range goals
         b. monthly calendars for short-range goals

      ii. organizer notebooks and systems (such as Daytimer and Covey system)
         a. develop daily lists and categorize priorities—most crucial actions first
         b. develop a list of high-peak (most essential) and low-peak (routine) activities
         c schedule most important tasks for part of the day when you work best

      iii. electronic organizers
         a. allow storage and retrieval of more data
         b. can eliminate repetition (calendar, address book, phone list)

      iv. note that paper or electronic organizers are tools—the nurse leader still requires an effective underlying time-management strategy, and that backing up data to protect against data loss is essential

(also see: Delegation: Chapter 20)

Questions

1. Which of the following is a characteristic of decision-making?
   a. it only involves logical, rational thought
   b. it is often the result of many incremental steps rather than one large step
   c. it must always be done quickly in a health care setting
   d. it is done from the top-down

2. Which of the following is true about effective critical thinkers?
   a. they seldom generate new ideas and alternatives
   b. they often say, "We've always done it this way, so let's do it this way again"
   c. they tend to analyze the components of a problem
   d. they generally do not assume another person's point of view

3. Which of the following is a strategic step in the decision-making process?
   a. maximax approach
   b. brainstorming session
   c. Delphi group
   d. determining goals

4. The likelihood that something will occur is called
   a. risk
   b. the Pareto principle
   c. maximax approach
   d. probability

5. A visual decision-making tool that graphically illustrates a project from start to finish is called
   a. decision tree
   b. PERT flowchart
   c. Gantt chart
   d. electronic organizer

6. In group decision-making, consensus means
   a. all group members can live with and support the decision
   b. members are not required to meet face to face
   c. all group members agree to think alike, no matter what the evidence
   d. the group uses the Delphi technique

7. A critical outcome deals with activities that are
   a. essential for patient safety and care
   b. life threatening or potentially life threatening

  c. needed to complete the plan of care

  d. essential for determining staffing of shifts to provide patient care

8. Which of the following is an effective way of keeping a meeting on track?

  a. send an agenda after the meeting

  b. avoid setting meeting time limits as they decrease attendees' creativity

  c. start and stop on time

  d. encourage full discussion so as to avoid follow-up meetings

9. Which of the following is a strategy for using downtime effectively?

  a. arrive 10 minutes early for all appointments

  b. call ahead to verify appointments

  c. avoid carrying reading materials around as they are heavy and slow you down

  d. return phone calls only from the privacy of your office

Critical Thinking Questions

1. A patient comes to the hospital outpatient center saying that he thinks he has been exposed to anthrax. He said he was paying a toll at the bridge, and when he checked his wallet later, noticed a white powder on his money. He is anxious and pacing, and talking rapidly. Using the decision-making tools described in this chapter, choose a condition of decision-making, a method for deciding how this situation should be handled and a plan for managing the situation.

2. Time management is a challenge for new graduates from nursing school when they take their first job. Interview a nurse with less than a year's experience, one with 3 to 5 years experience, one with 6 to 8 years experience and one with 10 or more years experience, Ask them what their experience has been with managing an assignment through prioritizing care and other time management strategies.

3. From the interviews above, compare how the interviews subjects' responses compare with Patricia Benner's levels of practice in *From Novice to Expert (1984)*. Do the interview subjects' responses correspond with Benner's findings?

Discussion Questions

1. Think of a person in your organization and analyze how that person makes decisions. What strategy or strategies does that person employ?

2. Evaluate how groups of people in your organization make decisions. Do they use consensus? Have they become involved in "groupthink"?

3. Who is the most effective time manager in your organization? What skills or strategies does he or she use to manage time?

4. What time management skills or strategies mentioned above do you use in your work or personal life? Why are they effective?

Works Cited

Benner, P. (1984). *From novice to expert: Excellence and power in clinical nursing practice.* Menlo Park, CA: Addison-Wesley Publishing.

Costello-Nickitas, D. (1997). *Quick reference to nursing leadership.* Clifton Park, NY: Thomson Delmar Learning.

Hansten, R. I., & Washburn, M. J. (1998). *Clinical delegation skills: A handbook for professional practice.* Gaithersburg, MD: Aspen.

Little-Stoetzel, S. (2003). Decision making. In P. Kelly-Heidenthal (Ed.), *Nursing leadership & management* (pp. 428–445). Clifton Park, NY: Thomson Delmar Learning.

Maloney, P. L. (2003). Time management. In P. Kelly-Heidenthal (Ed.), *Nursing leadership & management* (pp. 361–375). Clifton Park, NY: Thomson Delmar Learning.

Sullivan, E. J., & Decker, P. J. (1992). *Effective management in nursing* (3rd ed.). Redwood City, CA: Addison-Wesley Publishing.

Sullivan, E. J., & Decker, P. J. (2001). *Effective leadership and management in nursing* (5th ed.). Upper Saddle River, N.J.: Prentice Hall.

Upenieks, V. B. (1998). Work sampling: Assessing nursing efficiency. *Nursing Management, 49*(4), 27–29.

Urden, L., & Roode, J. (1997). Work sampling: A decision-making tool for determining resources and work design. *Journal of Nursing Administration, 27*(9), 34–41.

Additional Resources

Bly, R. W. (1999). *101 ways to make every second count: Time management tips and techniques for more success with less stress.* New York: Career Press.

Covey, S. (1989). *The seven habits of highly effective people.* New York: Simon and Schuster.

Duchscher, J. (1999). Catching the wave: Understanding the concept of critical thinking. *Journal of Advanced Nursing, 29*(3), 577–583.

Pratt, J. (2000). Time management: The hurrier I go, the behinder I get. *Home Health Care Management and Practice, 12*(4), 61.

O'Neill, E. S., Dluhy, N. M., Fortier, P. J., & Michel, H. E. (2004). Knowledge acquisition, synthesis, and validation: A model for decision support systems. *Journal of Advanced Nursing, 47*(2), 134-143.

Web-Based Calendars. (2001). *Training and Development, 55*(9), 29.

Web Sites

Barriers to Effective Clinical Decision Making in Nursing
 http://www.clininfo.health.nsw.gov.au/hospolic/stvincents/1993/a04.html

Brainstorming, Decision-making, and Time-management tools
 www.MindTools.com

Brainstorming Web
 http://www.graphic.org/brainst.html

Decision-Making for the Clinical Nurse
 http://www.nurseweek.com/ce/ce410a.html

National Association of Professional Organizers
 www.napo.net

Ohio State Board of Nursing Scope of Practice Decision Tool
 http://www.nursing.ohio.gov/pdfs/Decmodel.pdf

Time Management for Nurse Educators
 http://www.bcsnsg.org.uk/itin08/lewis.htm

Time Management for Student Nurses
 http://www.student-nurse.fsnet.co.uk/timetips.htm

Time Management in Patient Care
 http://www.graduateresearch.com/NavuTime.htm

CHAPTER 9

CHANGE MANAGEMENT SKILLS

INTRODUCTION

Nurse leaders are often called upon to be change agents who see the need for change, assess how it can be done, and deal effectively with the normal human resistance that always seems to accompany change. This chapter reviews what change is, theories about how change occurs, and strategies for effectively implementing change in organizations.

KEY POINTS

1. Definition

    A. **Change** is "the process of making something different from what it was" (Sullivan & Decker, 2001, p. 249)

        i. different actions are performed to achieve outcomes
        ii. goals or outcomes may or may not change
        iii. most changes are implemented for positive reasons (to improve patient care, efficiency, accuracy)
        iv. most organizational changes are planned and purposeful

B. Types of change

    i. **personal change**
       a. made voluntarily for an individual's particular reasons
       b. for example, a nurse moves to a smaller hospital setting to decrease stress and work day instead of night hours or a nurse changes work setting to become a telephone triage nurse after sustaining a back injury while lifting patients in a long-term care facility

    ii. **professional change**
       a. voluntarily and planned change in a job position or obtaining credentials (training or education), to further an individual's career goals
       b. for example, a nurse seeking professional change may take a nursing certification examination or choose to work in a different specialty area for professional development

    iii. **organizational change**
       a. planned change undertaken to improve outcomes, efficiency, financial standing, or to meet some other organizational goal
       b. changes in organizations may take employees by surprise if plans are not clearly communicated
       c. for example, an organization decides to move all nurses from eight-hour to twelve-hour shifts. This is a major operational change and those affected need to be informed about and included in the change process.
       d. organizational change that is not handled well causes an increase in staff stress and resistance and often mistrust of management (Sebastian, 1999; Anderson, 2003)

2. Nurses often act as **change agents** (one who is responsible for bringing about change)

A. In institutions

    i. nurses are most significant determiners of the length of patient stay in hospitals
    ii. nurse expertise and organizational skills determine cost and quality of care provided
    iii. nursing is the largest part of any organization's personnel budget
    iv. organizations known for outstanding nursing care have a competitive advantage in the health care marketplace

B. Outside institutions

    i. nurse change agents help move the health care system from a medical to a nursing model
    ii. promote healthy living

     iii. develop and manage prevention programs
     iv. create quality, cost-effective care for a wide range of patient populations
     v. provide case management services for most efficient use of technology and other resources
     vi. fill service gaps after people leave institutions
     vii. work as advocates for underserved populations (Sullivan & Decker, 1992)

  C. Entrepreneurial role of nurse change agent

     i. entrepreneurial nurses see change as healthy
     ii. characteristics of entrepreneur nurse include imagination, ingenuity, and persistence (Baumal, 1993)
     iii. changes in nursing roles resulting from entrepreneurial change include advanced practice nursing, case management, critical paths, and other professional practice models (Sullivan & Decker, 2001)

3. Change in nursing environments

  A. According to Marquis and Huston (2000), there are three basic reasons to introduce change:

     i. solve a problem; for example, inadequate staffing of RNs for a hospital's weekend or holiday shifts
     ii. improve efficiency; for example, provide care for postoperative patients using the most cost-effective mix of credentialed and noncredentialed care providers
     iii. reduce unnecessary workload on a person or group, for example, to ensure that an RN on the 3–11 p.m. shift is supervising no more than a certain number of assistive staff

  B. Other reasons why change occurs in the nursing environment

     i. technology. Automation for patient recordkeeping, billing, and diagnostics is constantly changing and becoming more networked. Although few organizations are completely "paperless," the trend is toward more, not less, technology.
     ii. changes in corporate structures. Restructuring is an ongoing activity, as organizations try to survive changing demands and markets by adding, expanding, or reducing services.
     iii. reimbursement. Pressure from payors and others, such as governments to control spending by emphasizing preventive care and less expensive outpatient vs. more costly inpatient services.
     iv. advances in treatments and medications. Increasing emphasis on preventive treatments, community health initiatives, outpatient

services, ambulatory surgery centers to meet patient care needs most effectively while controlling cost.

v. biomedical discoveries. Stem cell research, genetic therapies that can cure disease and improve quality of life (Sullivan & Decker, 1992)

4. Change agent characteristics and strategies

A. Successful change agents demonstrate certain characteristics. According to Sullivan & Decker (2001), a change agent must perceive that the current situation is unacceptable and understand how both the current situation and any possible change will affect all stakeholders. In addition, effective change agents tend to have most of the following characteristics, all of which can be cultivated and practiced.

   i.   ability to combine ideas from a variety of unconnected sources
   ii. ability to energize and motivate others
   iii. well-developed interpersonal skills, including group management and problem-solving skills
   iv. ability to work with system details while keeping the "big picture" in mind
   v.   a balance of flexibility and persistence—effective change agents are open-minded enough to see when they need to change, but are persistent enough to stick with their ideas in the face of nonproductive resistance from others
   vi. confident and not easily discouraged
   vii. ability to think realistically and strategically
   viii. ability to inspire others' trust in them; often occurs due to a history of integrity and success with other change efforts
   ix. ability to articulate ideas and vision
   x.   ability to handle resistance from those who oppose change

B. Change agent strategies. According to the classic model developed by Bennis, Benne, and Chinn (1969), three strategies can be used to facilitate change, depending on the amount of resistance and the characteristics of the change agent.

   i. **power-coercive**
       a. application of power by legitimate authority, such as law, policy, or financial appropriations
       b. people in control enforce changes; those not in power may not even be aware that changes are occurring and, even if aware, have little or no power to alter the course of change
       c. leadership response to resistance: accept it or leave it
       d. used when high levels of resistance are expected, change is critical, time is short, and there may be little or no chance of securing organizational consensus

    e. an example is the government's change in payment for patient care based on a diagnosis-related group (DRG) rather than costs

  ii. **empirical-rational**

    a. knowledge is the most powerful element for change

    b. this model assumes that people are rational and will act in their own self-interest, when that self-interest is made clear to them

    c. assumes that the change agent is able to persuade people that changes will benefit them

    d. effective when there is little resistance to change and the change is perceived as reasonable or beneficial

    e. this model could effectively be used to implement a technology change; for example, having nurses use PDAs to track procedure scheduling in an outpatient surgical setting. The change agent's job would be to explain the benefits to staff and patients of such a system as well as to provide appropriate training and backup, to further decrease any resistance.

  iii. **normative-reeducative**

    a. assumes that people act in accordance with social norms and values, and that they are less likely to change, based on information and rational arguments

    b. change agent focuses on people's behavioral motivators—such as roles, relationships, attitudes, and feelings—rather than rational motivators

    c. emphasis is not on persuasion but on interpersonal relationships between the change agent and the people he or she is influencing to change

    d. seen as an effective way to implement change in a health care environment

    e. effective for starting new services, for example, a postsurgical follow-up team, or to make systemic changes, for example, changing from inpatient to ambulatory surgical programs

5. Theories of change. Theories about how change occurs fall into two categories: **linear change theories** (assumes that change occurs in a stepwise, logical way) and **nonlinear change theories** (assumes that change is more chaotic than controlled).

  A. Traditional (linear) change theories include:

    i. Lewin's Force-Field Model (1951), which is made up of three steps:

      a. unfreezing: the old or usual way of doing things in an organization begins to change or "thaw" as people become aware that change needs to happen

    b. moving to a new level: change is introduced to and implemented in the organization; those affected by the change learn its benefits and disadvantages

    c. refreezing: the change or new way of operation becomes the norm and is incorporated into people's habits or routines

  ii. Lippitt's Phases of Change (Lippitt, Watson, & Westley, 1958). Derived from Lewin's model but defines seven total steps in the change process.

    a. diagnose the problem: for example, inadequate supervision of assistive staff

    b. assess motivation and capacity for change: does the staff want to be more closely supervised; is an RN available and willing to take on this challenge?

    c. assess change agent's motivation and resources: does the RN have excellent organizational and communication skills? Is he or she motivated by the desire to improve how patient care is delivered (as opposed to "doing supervision" to avoid other job responsibilities)?

    d. select appropriate progressive change objectives: for example, in the next month, assign all staff to a mentor, institute weekly meetings of noncredentialed personnel, and arrange for the supervisory RN to complete a "managing difficult people" course

    e. choose appropriate role for change agent: for example, mentor, facilitator (rather than "criticizer" or "enforcer")

    f. maintain the change once it has started: provide logistical support to meet the RN's needs to continue to act as a change agent; provide a feedback forum for the assistive staff

    g. terminate the helping relationship: once the change is instituted and has become the norm, no need to supervise the supervisor or otherwise oversee his or her staff

  iii. Havelock's six-step model. Like Lippitt's model, this is based on Lewin's model, but breaks the change process into additional steps. The first three steps are the planning stage and the last three steps are referred to as the moving stage. Havelock (1973) particularly emphasized the essential role of planning in any change endeavor.

    a. build a relationship: people affected by the change need to be involved in it, and this occurs through building relationships in the organization

    b. diagnose the problem

    c. acquire resources. gather the money, technology, staff, etc. needed to successfully implement the change

    d. choose the solution

     e. gain acceptance for the solution: Havelock believed that this step would occur only if the first step (building relationships) had occurred

     f. stabilize and self-renewal: organization functions on the new level; change becomes part of the norm and the organization enjoys the benefits of the change

  iv. Rogers' Diffusion of Innovations theory (1983). Rogers' theory emphasizes the changeability of change itself—and that efforts to implement change may be rejected at first, then later accepted. The initial rejection is not the final word. This method involves a five-step process of innovation and decision-making.

     a. knowledge: people who can make the decision are introduced to the change and begin to understand it. For example, a home care agency begins to learn about telemonitoring technology for patients with congestive heart failure.

     b. persuasion: people form a favorable (or unfavorable) attitude about the change. For example, some nurses discuss how the technology saves travel time, while others express their frustration with computer compatibility problems in the field. After a time, a general perception forms (such as: "there are glitches but the system works overall" or "the technology is flawed and increases our workload").

     c. decision: people engage in various activities that lead to a decision to either adopt or reject the change. For example, nurses with more computer experience mentor others in troubleshooting; supervisors call all nurses using the telemonitoring technology, and have them fill out a survey that rates their satisfaction or dissatisfaction about the telemonitoring program. Supervisors then solicit specific feedback that can guide modifications when necessary.

     d. implementation: the change is put into action; at this stage, the change maybe adapted to better fit the situation. For example, the home care staff may decide to add an autorecord feature to a blood pressure monitor, to compensate for inaccurate reporting by visually impaired patients.

     e. confirmation: decision makers seek reinforcement that their decision was correct; conflicting feedback might result in the decision being reversed or modified. For example, home care nurses look for data that confirm that the technology benefited both patients (avoiding rehospitalization) and nurses (less travel, quicker response time).

B. Nonlinear change theories

  i. **chaos theory.** This theory, developed by Thietart and Forgues (1995) says that

      a. most organizations have the potential to be chaotic

      b. this chaos actually has a underlying order

      c. organizations often undergo a series of rapid changes, and stabilize until the next round of rapid changes occurs

      d. leadership in these organizations must be flexible and able to respond quickly and appropriately to the rapid changes

    ii. **learning organization theory.** This theory, developed by Peter Senge (1990), emphasizes the systemic interdependence of organizations. According to Senge, learning organizations:

      a. are flexible and responsive

      b. act as open systems

      c. are interdependent (and understand that if a part does not work well, the whole will not work either)

      d. share five traits: systems thinking, personal mastery, mental models, shared vision, and team learning

      e. are able to "sort out" chaos and respond appropriately to it (Sullivan & Decker, 2001; Anderson, 2003)

C. Theories about reactions to change. Bushy (1992) identified six behaviors that people exhibit in response to change:

    i. innovators: people who enjoy the challenge that change brings and often instigate or implement change

    ii. early adopters: open to change; will work with change that is brought to them but are not as change-focused as the innovators

    iii. early majority: people who enjoy the status quo but who will adopt change earlier than average, to avoid being left behind

    iv. later majority: slower to adopt change; often express reluctance about or skepticism of change efforts

    v. laggards: last people to adopt a change; may be suspicious of change; prefer stability and tradition

    vi. rejectors: people who openly oppose or reject change; they maybe direct or indirect in their resistance

6. The change process consists of the following six steps. Note the relation between change process and nursing process.

A. Assessment

    i. identify problem or opportunity

    ii. collect or analyze data about change

    iii. data are derived from both internal and external sources

    iv. data analysis should support both the need for change and the potential action selected

    v. set goals for what the change shall accomplish

B. Planning
   i. determine who will be affected by change and when change will occur
   ii. examine all potential actions
   iii. should include how change will be implemented
   iv. construct an evaluation component to assess if the change met the original goals for the change

C. Implementation. Most organizations use one of three strategies for promoting change (see above for more details):

   i. power-coercive: based on power, authority, and control of change agent; low participation from those the change will impact
   ii. normative-reeducative: emphasis on using group norms to socialize individuals; because people want to maintain relationships in the organization, they will go along with the change
   iii. rational-empirical: people are rational (thinking) beings and will use knowledge and logic to adapt to change; people who are taught the advantages of change will readily accept it

E. Evaluation

   i. determines if change is effective, based on outcomes (goals) identified during assessment and using the evaluation method established during planning
   ii. many organizations overlook this step, but it is very important, just as in nursing process, so that modifications can be made when needed
   iii. needs to be properly timed (not too early before changes have stabilized, and not too late, after change has become "old news" and the "new normal")

F. Stabilization

   i. using policies and procedures, for example, to make change the norm rather than the innovation
   ii. should occur as soon as possible, to complete the change process (Anderson, 2003)

G. Becoming a change agent. How is being a change agent being a leader?

   i. change agents and leaders manage the dynamics of change
   ii. change agents and leaders are able to maintain a vision of the organization, the ongoing change, and the organization's goals
   iii. change agents and leaders know the organization, the change process, and the people involved

      iv. change agents and leaders communicate effectively and proactively with all affected people throughout the change process

      v. change agents and leaders have integrity and are respected and trusted by others

7. Communication plan for facilitating change. According to Costello-Nickitas (1997), change leaders must have an effective plan for communicating essential information about change. An effective communication plan includes the following components:

  A. Adequate resources

      i. telephone, bulletin boards, e-mail, newsletters, Internet, and/or intranet

      ii. messages should be sent to everyone involved in or affected by the change

  B. Choose appropriate format

      i. generally simple, unified messages are best

      ii. may be memo, e-mail, or other mode, depending on the needs of the particular organization and the members who need to learn about the change

  C. Invest in targeted face-to-face meetings.

      i. meetings augment written messages

      ii. provide people a chance to give feedback and two-way communication

      iii. should occur every two to three weeks during an ongoing change effort

  D. Strategies that change agents can use to manage change. According to Anderson (2003), change agents can manage the change process using these strategies:

      i. articulate vision

         a. use the same key words for all discussions about the change

         b. constantly remind people of the goals and vision—the positive things that will come as a result of the change

      ii. map out a timeline for the change and the steps required

      iii. plant the seeds

         a. talk to key people in the organization about what will happen or what is expected; use and repeat key words or core message(s)

         b. information will quickly filter through the rest of the organization

  iv. carefully select the change project team, making sure that
    a. stakeholders are strongly represented
    b. there are sufficient experts to evaluate the change
    c. people who are expected to resist change are also included
  v. create consistency
    a. set and keep meeting dates
    b. use timeline to stay on track with change process activities
  vi. provide regular updates
    a. in writing
    b. to supervisors, peers, and subordinates
  vii. deal with conflict directly
    a. check out rumors; it is essential for change agent leaders to tap into the "grapevine"—the informal communication structure of any organization. Even if information being passed on the grapevine is incorrect, it establishes a reality for many of those who will be affected by change.
    b. do not seek conflict, do not ignore it either
  viii. maintain a positive attitude, and avoid getting discouraged in the face of resistance
  ix. be aware of political forces at work
    a. get consensus on key actions as the change process progresses, especially for issues of policy, finance, or operating philosophy
    b. recognize barriers that arise and work to get consensus to overcome them
  x. know who the leaders are
    a. recognize both formal and informal leaders
    b. create a relationship with them and consult them regularly
  xi. maintain self-confidence and foster trust with others.

E. Additional ways to facilitate change. According to Costello-Nickitas (1997), effective change agents also use the following actions to facilitate change:

  i. recognize and respond to the impact of change on people
    a. avoid arguing with people about their feelings regarding change, and avoid telling them that "it isn't so bad;" support the need for change with facts that are important to people unsettled by the change taking place
    b. acknowledge with empathy that people are often unsettled by changes
  ii. use communication skills to help people process the impacts of change.
    a. give people a chance to talk through their feelings
    b. use conversations to provide information about the change—who, what, when, where, why, how

      c. repeat the message. Use the "7 × 7 rule" of saying a message seven different times in seven different ways

   iii. anticipate grief

      a. people undergoing change often experience grief stages (shock, denial, anger, bargaining, anxiety, and sadness)

      b. openly recognize that even positive change can mean the loss of a valued way of doing things, and that grief may occur

   iv. acknowledge period of confusion, when people maybe confused or unhappy about the changes that are occurring

   v. expect resistance, a natural reaction to change

REVIEW ACTIVITIES

Questions

1. A voluntarily and planned change in a job position or obtaining credentials such as training or education is an example of:

  a. personal change
  b. professional change
  c. organizational change
  d. resistance to change

2. When people in control enforce changes in an organization and others in the organization have no input into these changes, this is an example of which of the following change strategies?

  a. normative-reeducative
  b. power-coercive
  c. change-stabilization
  d. rational-empirical

3. The change strategy that assumes that people act more in accordance with social values and are less likely to change based on information or rational arguments is called the:

  a. stabilization-evaluation strategy
  b. power-coercive strategy
  c. normative-reeducative strategy
  d. rational-empirical strategy

4. Unfreezing, moving to a new level, and refreezing are steps that make up which of the following theories/models of change?

  a. Lewin's Force-Field Model
  b. Lippitt's Phases of Change

    c.   Havelock's Six-Step Change Model

    d.   Rogers' Diffusion of Innovations

5. According to this change theory, efforts to implement change may be rejected at first and accepted later; thus an initial rejection is not the final word. Which theory is this?

    a.   Lewin's Force-field Model

    b.   Lippitt's Phases of Change

    c.   Havelock's Six-Step Change Model

    d.   Rogers' Diffusion of Innovations

6. This theory says that organizations often undergo a series of rapid changes, and then stabilize until the next round of rapid changes occurs.

    a.   Lippitt's Phases of Change theory

    b.   Havelock's Six-Step Change theory

    c.   chaos theory

    d.   learning organization theory

7. In Bushy's theory about people's reaction to change, the people who enjoy the status quo but who will adopt change earlier than average to avoid being left behind are called:

    a.   innovators

    b.   laggards

    c.   early majority

    d.   early adopters

8. Identifying the problem or opportunity and collecting or analyzing data about a possible change are activities of which step of the change process?

    a.   assessment

    b.   planning

    c.   implementation

    d.   stabilization

9. The final step needed to complete the change process is called:

    a.   assessment

    b.   planning

    c.   implementation

    d.   stabilization

10. The "7 × 7 rule" of communicating a message about change means:

    a.   send the message seven different times in seven different ways

    b.   all memos should be 7 × 7 inches

    c.   there should be no more than 49 messages in any change process

    d.   send seven messages a day for seven days

Critical Thinking Questions

1. Change is a key aspect of nursing practice. Adopting evidence-based practice is one way of supporting change in an organization.
   a. Define evidence-based practice.
   b. One area of debate in clinical practice is about which dressing is most appropriate for pressure ulcers and which wound care protocol is most effective. Review the nursing literature on this issue to determine what approach is supported by research. Then, choose one of the change theories outlined in this chapter and describe how you would implement the steps of that approach to change practice in your local hospital from "traditional" practice to evidence-based practice in this area. How will you make the case and implement the change? Do not forget to analyze the organizational culture and plan your change strategy accordingly.

2. Many hospitals have been forced to close in-patient units and merge units because of reduced in-patient census and lower reimbursement rates from third-party payors. Assume that you are the leader of an orthopedic nursing unit that is being closed and merged with a general surgery unit in the same hospital. How would you approach this merger and manage this change? Choose one of the change theories outlined in this chapter as the rationale for your actions.

3. You have been asked to be a part of the team that implements a change from your old computer system to a new patient tracking software that uses laptops and PDAs. Using the models above, sketch out an effective communication plan to help implement this change.

Discussion Questions

1. Think of a significant change that occurred in your organization within the past year. How was the change implemented? Who were the change leaders? What method of change leadership did they use?

2. Think of another change in which you have been involved. Was it handled well or poorly? What was wrong, or what contributed to the success of implementing this change? How would you have done things differently?

3. What kind of behavioral response do you tend to have to change? Using Bushy's categories, find the response that best fits and name one behavior that places you in that category.

Works Cited

Anderson, M. M. (2003). Change and conflict resolution. In P. Kelly-Heidenthal (Ed.), *Nursing leadership & management* (pp. 326–345). Clifton Park, NY: Thomson Delmar Learning.

Baumal, W. J. (1993). *Entrepreneurship, management, and the structure of payoffs.* London: MIT Press.

Bennis, W., Benne, K., & Chinn, R. (Eds.). (1969). *The planning of change* (2nd ed.). New York: Holt, Rinehart & Winston.

Bushy, A. (1993). Managing change: Strategies for continuing education. *The Journal of Continuing Education in Nursing, 23,* 197–200.

Costello-Nickitas, D. (1997). *Quick reference to nursing leadership.* Clifton Park, NY: Thomson Delmar Learning.

Havelock, R. G. (1973). *The change agent's guide to innovation in education.* Englewood Cliffs, NJ: Educational Technology.

Lewin, K. (1951). *Field theory in social science.* New York: Harper & Row.

Lippitt, R., Watson, J., & Westley, B. (1958). *The dynamics of planned change.* New York: Harcourt, Brace and World.

Marquis, B. L., & Huston, C. J. (2000). *Leadership roles and management functions in nursing: Theory applied* (3rd ed.). Philadelphia: Lippincott.

Rogers, E. (1983). *Diffusion of innovations* (3rd ed.). New York: Free Press.

Sebastian, J. G. (1999). Organizational change and the change process. In J. Lancaster, *Nursing issues in leading and managing change.* St. Louis, MO: Mosby.

Senge, P. (1990). *The fifth discipline: The art and practice of the learning organization.* New York: Doubleday.

Sullivan, E. J., & Decker, P. J. (1992). *Effective management in nursing* (3rd ed.). Redwood City, CA: Addison-Wesley Publishing.

Sullivan, E. J., & Decker, P. J. (2001). *Effective leadership and management in nursing* (5th ed.). Upper Saddle River, N.J.: Prentice Hall.

Theitart, R. A., & Forgues, B. (1995). Chaos theory and organizations. *Organization Science, 6*(1), 19–31.

Additional References

Bennett, M. (2003). The manager as agent of change. *Nursing Management, 10*(7), 20–24.

Jooste, K. (2004). Leadership: A new perspective. *Journal of Nursing Management, 12*(3), 217–224.

Kaminski, J. Leadership and change management: Navigating the turbulent frontier. Available at http://www.nursing-informatics.com/changemant.html

Ortner, P. M. (2004). The nurse as change agent: An approach to environmental health advocacy training. *Policy, Politics & Nursing Practice, 5*(2), 125–131.

Todd, J. (2003). Do you have change agents on your staff? *Nursing Homes Long Term Care Management, 52*(8), 33–36.

Web Sites

Change: University of North Florida
http://www.unf.edu/~lloriz/change.htm

Change Agents Home Page
http://www.dhutton.com/change

Change Management: Change Without Migraines Resources
http://www.beyondresistance.com/htm/2articles.html

Change Management: Reducing Surgical Site Infections
http://www.gehealthcare.com/prod_sol/hcare/pdf/CAMC_PSQH.PDF

Change Management Resource Library
http://www.change-management.org/articles.htm

Health and Social Care Change Agent Team
http://www.changeagentteam.org.uk/

Health Plan as Change Agent: Health Management Technology
http://www.healthmgttech.com/archives/0904/0904the_health_plan.htm

CONFLICT RESOLUTION SKILLS

KEY TERMS

accommodating

avoiding

collaborating

competing

compromising

conflict

conflict resolution methods

confronting

disagreement

dysfunctional conflict

intrapersonal conflict

interpersonal conflict

negotiating

organizational conflict

INTRODUCTION

Nurse leaders must deal with the constant change that is now a normal part of working in health care. However, with change comes conflict—the differences in values, goals, or actions between people or groups of people. Effective nurse leaders must recognize the benefits of conflict and learn ways to manage it effectively so that conflict can result in organizational and personal growth.

KEY POINTS

1. Definition

    A. **Conflict** is the "consequence of real or perceived differences in mutually exclusive goals, values, ideas, attitudes, beliefs, feelings, or actions" (Sullivan & Decker, 2001, p. 185).

    B. Conflict is a common and important part of the change process:

        i. change highlights differences in values, beliefs, or actions

        ii. conflict, however, is not automatically negative

     iii. conflict can allow for creativity and innovation as well as encourage productive discussions of varying points of view

C.   Difference between disagreement and conflict

     i. **disagreement** is like a "mini" conflict; it may be based on interpersonal, cultural, logistical, or other differences
     ii. some disagreements can grow into conflicts but not all do
     iii. astute leaders try to determine which disagreements have the potential to become conflicts and attempt to address them before conflict grows

D.   Dysfunctional conflict. According to Costello-Nickitas (1997) **dysfunctional conflict**

     i. is disruptive and counterproductive; for example, dysfunctional conflict often takes organizational issues and turns them into personal issues or attacks
     ii. destroys group process, trust, and other important functions in an organization
     iii. challenge for nurse leaders who have to
        a. simultaneously manage the group creating the dysfunctional conflict and let the group know it is not handling the situation appropriately and
        b. support the group members as individuals and avoid creating a climate intolerant to conflict of any sort

E.   Other components that affect how people perceive and handle conflict

     i. personality
        a. preferred communication style
        b. whether a person prefers to engage in or avoid conflict
        c. level of tolerance for multiple or competing perspectives
        d. partly a result of inborn traits and partly a result of learned (usually familial) behaviors
     ii. training
        a. communication skills
        b. conflict assessment and management
        c. psychology and human behavior
        d. organizational dynamics
     iii. culture
        a. of the person: whether they are more conflict tolerant or have been acculturated to avoid conflict
        b. of the organization: whether an organization sees conflict as having value or whether it is perceived as negative and/or destructive (Anderson, 2003)

F. According to Marquis and Huston (2000), effective nurse leaders facilitate conflict resolution, regardless of management role, by engaging in the following actions:

    i. model conflict resolution methods when conflict is noted

        a. this demonstrates awareness (does not ignore conflict or try to make it "go away")

        b. this sets up conflict as a resolvable situation that all parties can win

        c. for example, a nurse leader can choose to set up meetings or discussions that allow all parties to be heard

    ii. help conflicted parties identify techniques that can resolve the conflict

        a. a key technique is fostering open and honest communication

        b. effective conflict managers are nonjudgmental about differences and avoid accusing either side

        c. for example, a nurse leader dealing with a conflict between two senior nurses will avoid taking sides and will not discuss the nurses or their conflict with others

    iii. create an environment that is conducive to resolving conflict

        a. a nurse leader uses authority (formal or informal) in a positive and strategic way

        b. for example, if there is a conflict between the financial office and the nurses on a unit concerning completing paperwork so that all charges are captured, nurse leaders can use their authority to ensure that all information is available, that nurses have access to appropriate training, and that sufficient resources are allocated to meet both financial compliance and patient care goals

2. Types of conflict. According to Anderson (2003), there are three broad categories of conflict.

A. **Intrapersonal**

    i. occurs within the individual

    ii. for example, a nurse leader can experience internal conflict about whether to stay in her current position, which he likes, or to move to a higher-level position, which has a much higher pay rate but also more stress and less flexible hours

B. **Interpersonal**

    i. occurs between people, groups, or work teams

    ii. may involve a disagreement about values or philosophy

    iii. often is due to differing or incompatible personalities or work styles

iv. for example, a newly hired nurse begins to press for updating a computer system based on her previous experience; nurses who have used and are comfortable with the current system do not see sufficient reason to change

C. **Organizational**

   i. occurs within organizations
   ii. is a result of scarce resources, cultural differences, or changes in infrastructure
   iii. often reflects departmental differences in values and philosophies
   iv. for example, the financial department of a rehabilitation hospital requires certain key input to ensure that all charge items are captured; nurses on the units say that the coding is confusing and that they spend precious patient care time "filling in forms"
   v. in many conflict situations, conflicts such as the above can help organizations identify areas for improvement. In this scenario, both financial accountability and patient care are important and how the conflict is handled should address both sides.

3. People use a number of different methods to resolve conflict. Some are more useful or desirable than others, although, depending on the conflict and situation, each method may have some use. Following are the most common **conflict resolution methods** and advantages and disadvantages of each.

A. **Avoiding.** This is perhaps the most common technique that people use. When people avoid conflict, they ignore it—either consciously (by refusing to engage) or unconsciously (by denying that a conflict exists).

   i. advantages
      a. may enable people to avoid turning minor disagreements into larger conflicts
      b. does not overreact to a situation
   ii. disadvantages
      a. through avoiding, a person could be ignoring an issue that needs to be dealt with
      b. conflicts can sometimes escalate because they are not being dealt with
      c. conflict avoiders risk being left out of the loop concerning changes and innovations

B. **Accommodating.** This conflict resolution method, also called smoothing or cooperating, is used when a person ignores his or her own feelings about an issue in order to agree with (accommodate) the other side.

   i. advantages

      a. if an issue is relatively minor, accommodating allows the parties to move on to issues that are more important

      b. one side accommodating on one issue can make the other side more willing to accommodate on another issue

  ii. disadvantages

      a. can become a power struggle—with one side trying to get the other to "give in"

      b. more conflict rather than less can ensue if parties disagree about the importance of the issues being accommodated

      c. parties that consistently ignore their feelings and "give in" can wind up feeling frustrated or used, and maybe less willing to cooperate in the future

C. **Competing.** With this method, one side wins the conflict and the other side loses. It is sometimes called "forcing" because the winner forces the loser to accept his or her perspective on the conflict.

  i. advantages

      a. useful when an issue is critical or time to resolve the issue is limited

      b. can help move a critical but unpopular decision quickly through an organization

  ii. disadvantages

      a. losers tend to resent losing

      b. anger and resentment increases

      c. those on the losing side of the agreement may be less willing to engage in future conflicts or disagreements and may more regularly adopt a withdrawing or avoiding style

D. **Compromising.** With this method, each side gives up something as well as gets something. This method is used when both sides have a reasonable, important goal and losing is not required.

  i. advantages

      a. effective for interpersonal conflicts

      b. produces an "everybody wins something" scenario

      c. can be efficient method for resolving conflict when the issues have higher importance and there is limited time for resolution

  ii. disadvantages

      a. the winning and losing exchanges are seen as unfair or providing an advantage for one side

      b. conflict may resume if one side perceives that what it gave up was more important than the benefit received

      c. may not be as effective when one party is inherently less powerful than the other

E. **Negotiating.** This method is often defined as an extension of compromise, with higher stakes and more deliberate techniques to bargain for each side's give and take. Some experts (Lewicki, Hiam, & Olander, 1996) note that whether negotiating is more of a win-win, win-lose, or neutral (split the difference) situation depends on how much of a relationship the parties wish to continue after the negotiations are finished.

    i. advantages
        a. useful for high stakes issues
        b. solution usually seen as formal and more permanent than compromise
        c. does not require consensus
        d. conflict tends not to recur once the negotiations are finished
    ii. disadvantages
        a. getting to an agreement may be long and involved
        b. negotiations often seen as permanent, which can be a problem if one side decides that it is not satisfied with the results
        c. results maybe less satisfactory if one side feels that it has to give up too much to negotiate for what it wins

F. **Collaborating.** In this conflict resolution method, both sides in a conflict work to develop the outcome that is best for both sides. The emphasis is on creative problem solving so that each side meets its key goals.

    i. advantages
        a. seeks a permanent solution that achieves the goals and objectives of both parties
        b. is creative and allows parties to develop new solutions, rather than trading win/loss options
    ii. disadvantages
        a. may require significant resources, especially time
        b. requires that all parties are committed to success, possibly leaving the process open to interference by parties who do not want the conflict to have resolution
        c. requires that parties (and/or a facilitator) have significant creative, critical thinking, and problem-solving skills

G. **Confronting.** This method attempts to block the conflict from the start. This very powerful method brings the parties together, clarifies issues, and achieves an outcome.

    i. advantages
        a. prevents conflict from ever really developing
        b. powerful and decisive; no ambiguity
    ii. disadvantages
        a. can make a relatively minor conflict seem much more important than it is
        b. does not allow the positive aspects of conflict to develop
        c. can create an organizational climate of conflict intolerance (Anderson, 2003)

4. Dealing with difficult people. According to Costello-Nickitas (1997), facilitating conflict resolution often means dealing with difficult people who cause or worsen conflict. Every organization has them—they are negative, complain frequently, and generally seem to enjoy making other people unhappy. While a nurse leader may not be able to change a person's behavior, the leader can use techniques to offset the difficult person's influence. Following are typical "difficult people" behaviors and actions that can be used to deal effectively with them.

A.   Attackers

   i.   aggressive about stating their thoughts and feelings about all situations

   ii.   often demand that others listen to them while they ventilate their viewpoint

   iii.   may complain loudly that they are being ignored (or worse) if they feel they are not getting enough "ventilation time"

   iv.   effective nurse leader's actions

     a.   address person by name

     b.   speak quietly but firmly

     c.   encourage them to sit down and talk

     d.   remain calm while listening to them; speak slowly and deliberately to offset their aggressive tone and stance

B.   Egotists

   i.   self-centered

   ii.   expect others to listen to them

   iii.   often take on a "know it all" attitude

   iv.   make sure they are the center of attention (either as expert, or a clown or a distractor)

   v.   effective nurse leader's actions

     a.   is honest about and respectful of their abilities, but not intimidated by them

     b.   use them as resources

     c.   in a group, thank them for their contributions, then specifically ask other people in the group to contribute ("That's a great idea, Terry, thanks. Now let's hear from someone else. Chris, what do you think about this new protocol?")

C.   Sneaks

   i.   use sarcasm and criticism

   ii.   may be dishonest—saying one thing to a person and then doing another

   iii.   often set others up for failure

   iv.   effective nurse leader's actions

a. confront with questions that address their attitudes and behaviors
b. suggest positive ways to improve behavior
c. state clearly that sarcasm and dishonesty are not appropriate
d. encourage them to be a productive part of a team

D. Victims or chronic complainers

i. very negative worldview
ii. often act defeated, hopeless, and powerless
iii. try to get others to feel that way, as well
iv. effective nurse leader actions
   a. encourage them to express their viewpoints, and then question why they hold that particular perspective ("You say that this computer system will never work. Can you tell me more about which parts you see as nonfunctional?")
   b. use data to examine the situation and openly discuss whether the data and the person's perspective correspond
   c. offer resources and assistance when possible

E. Negators/nay-sayers

i. convinced that their way is the only way; anyone else's way of doing things is to be resisted
ii. most common response to a situation is "We can't do that. We've never done it before. It won't work."
iii. do not trust people in positions of authority
iv. often try to undermine authority figures
v. effective nurse leader's actions
   a. require a collective approach from the whole team, not just the leader. Have other team members offer suggestions and recommendations for solving problems
   b. encourage peer pressure to help the negator see other perspectives

F. Approval seekers

i. people who say "yes" to everything
ii. often agree to do work, then never complete it
iii. require a great deal of recognition and support
iv. effective nurse leader's actions
   a. acknowledge their efforts
   b. monitor work assignments and establish regular checkpoints, so that the person is never too far behind on a given task or project without the nurse leader being aware
   c. reward completed activities
   d. question the "yes" ("Thanks for agreeing to work on this policy committee, Alex. I appreciate that you're always looking

for ways to improve guidelines to help our department work more smoothly. But are you sure you want to take this on? You have two major report deadlines coming up in the next few weeks. I'm much more interested in your finishing those first, than maybe joining the policy committee later.")

G.   Withdrawers

    i.   keep to themselves and avoid participating

    ii.   rarely contribute to any group discussion or process

    iii.   may perform other tasks (doodling, checking cell phone voice mail, etc.) during meetings to avoid participation

    iv.   effective nurse leader's actions

        a.   actively engage unresponsive people by asking open-ended questions, directed specifically to them, "Jessie, what potential problems do you see with implementing this new scheduling plan?"

        b.   directly ask for their assistance on a task

        c.   pair the withdrawer and a more active participant who can serve as a mentor

5. Rules for effective conflict resolution. There are varieties of conflict resolution models, but all follow some basic rules. According to Sullivan and Decker (2001), using the following standards will make conflict resolution more likely to succeed.

A.   Protect each party's self-respect

    i.   deal with conflict

    ii.   avoid making the conflict a battle of personalities

B.   Do not blame the problem on the participants

    i.   blaming seldom accomplishes anything except making participants defensive

    ii.   instead, acknowledge that participants are responsible for developing a solution

C.   Allow all parties in the conflict to completely discuss their perspective of the problem, while maintaining focus on the problem and not on side or related issues that can easily get the discussion off-topic

D.   Set ground rules

    i.   establish the rules clearly before the discussions begin

    ii.   maintain equity in how often and how long each party presents its views

    iii.   ensure that parties of higher power or status do not take over the discussion; intervene, if necessary, to give lower status parties equal time for response

E. Encourage full expression

    i. provide an accepting atmosphere
    ii. allow parties to express both positive and negative feelings

F. Encourage active listening

    i. have one party summarize the contents of the other's statement before stating his or her own
    ii. discourage interrupting, answering, distracting, or other techniques that interfere with listening

G. Identify the key themes in the discussion (helps keep discussions on track)

    i. restate them at regular intervals and bring participants back to focus on the key elements as needed
    ii. ask parties in the discussion if they feel that key themes are being addressed

H. Encourage frequent feedback

    i. have participants restate the other's position
    ii. set aside specific time for responses and questions
    iii. provide a structure, if necessary, to facilitate feedback (for example, have participants give one "warm" or positive item of feedback and one "cool" or less positive item of feedback)

I. Help participants develop alternative solutions

    i. choose a mutually agreeable action
    ii. develop a plan to carry it out
    iii. make sure all parties agree to the solution (or are willing to accept it) and have sufficient resources to carry it out

J. Follow up on actions at an agreed-upon interval, and provide feedback to all participants

REVIEW ACTIVITIES

Questions

1. Which of the following is a true statement about conflict?
    a. it seldom occurs as part of the change process in health care settings
    b. it highlights differences in values, beliefs, or actions
    c. it is automatically negative
    d. it discourages creativity and innovation

2. Conflict that occurs between groups or teams is called:

    a. interpersonal
    b. intrapersonal
    c. organizational
    d. dysfunctional

3. In this conflict resolution method, a person ignores his or her own feelings about an issue in order to agree with the other side.

    a. collaborating
    b. confronting
    c. accommodating
    d. withdrawing

4. With this method of conflict resolution, each side gives up something as well as gets something.

    a. negotiating
    b. competing
    c. avoiding
    d. compromising

5. Difficult people who often demand that others listen to them while they ventilate their viewpoint are referred to as:

    a. attackers
    b. sneaks
    c. victims
    d. withdrawers

6. A person who readily agrees to do work, then never completes it may be a(n):

    a. approval seeker
    b. negator
    c. chronic complainer
    d. egotist

7. Which of the following would be an effective action to help resolve conflict?

    a. set ground rules
    b. discourage interruptions
    c. blame the problem on the participants
    d. limit feedback

Critical Thinking Questions

1. Conflicts that nurses encounter are not only with coworkers; two major issues of conflict for nurses in the clinical setting are conflicts with families and conflicts with physicians. Develop a plan for addressing conflict in each of these situations:

a. You are acting as charge nurse for the evening shift, when, at 8:30 p.m., an angry family member insists on talking with you. While the family member has a barrage of issues, they hinge on the fact that the staff nurse told the two visiting family members that visiting hours were over and that they had to leave. When they resisted, the nurse threatened to call security to enforce the rules. How can you handle this conflict?

b. You are in a patient's room talking with the patient, when you hear one of the general surgeons shouting, "Where the hell is a nurse when I need one? I don't have time to stand here and wait for somebody to get back from a coffee break to assist me!" How would you manage the conflict here?

Discussion Questions

1. Think of a conflict that has recently occurred (or is occurring) in school or at your clinical site or at your workplace. What kind of conflict is it? What are the different values, actions, or feelings of those who are having the conflict?

2. Think of an example of an interpersonal conflict you have recently encountered, and analyze your conflict resolution style. What method of conflict resolution do you tend to use? Is it effective or ineffective? Why? How might you make it more effective?

3. Everyone deals with difficult people. Think about a difficult person or people you have worked with. What are their characteristics and behaviors? How would you categorize them (negator, etc.)? Do you ever use these behaviors?

Works Cited

Anderson, M. M. (2003). Change and conflict resolution. In P. Kelly-Heidenthal (Ed.), *Nursing leadership & management* (pp. 326–345). Clifton Park, NY: Thomson Delmar Learning.

Costello-Nickitas, D. (1997). *Quick reference to nursing leadership.* Clifton Park, NY: Thomson Delmar Learning.

Lewicki, R. J., Hiam, A., & Olander, K. W. (1996). *Think before you speak.* New York: John Wiley & Sons.

Marquis, B. L., & Huston, C. J. (2000). *Leadership roles and management functions in nursing: Theory applied* (3rd ed.). Philadelphia: Lippincott.

Sullivan, E. J., & Decker, P. J. (2001). *Effective leadership and management in nursing* (5th ed.). Upper Saddle River, NJ: Prentice Hall.

Additional Resources

Brinkman, R., & Kirschner, R. (2002). *Dealing with people you can't stand: How to bring out the best in people at their worst.* New York: McGraw-Hill.

Building Collaboration Between ICU Nurses and Physicians. (2004). *American Journal of Nursing, 104*(6), 18.

Communication skills. (2003). Keeping conflict constructive: Empowering staff to improve care for seniors. *Care Connect, 18*(4), 20–21.

Deutsch, M., & Coleman, P. T. (Ed.) (2000). *Handbook of conflict resolution.* San Francisco: Jossey-Bass.

Johnson, S. (1998). *Who moved my cheese? An amazing way to deal with change in your work and life.* New York: Putnam.

Maxwell, M. (2004). HR Help for Religious Holiday Scheduling, Behavior Issues, and Turnover. *Nursing Economics, 22*(1), 39–41.

Porter O'Grady, T., & Epstein, D. G. (2003). When push comes to shove: Managers as mediators. *Nursing Management, 34*(10), 34–39.

Sitzman, K. (2004). A 10-step path for conflict resolution. *Home Healthcare Nurse, 22*(5), 335

Smith, S. B. (2001). Resolving conflict realistically in today's health care environment. *Journal of Psychosocial Nursing and Mental Health Services, 39*(11), 36–47.

Xu, Y. (2004). Conflict management styles of Asian and Asian American nurses: Implications for the nurse manager. *Health Care Manager, 23*(1), 46–53.

Web Sites

Association for Conflict Resolution
http://www.acrnet.org

Commitment to Workplace Advocacy Texas Nurses Association
http://www.texasnurses.org/wkplaceadv/commitments.htm

Conflict Resolution: Phyllis Beck Kritek
http://www.nurseweek.com/5min/kritek.html

Conflict Resolution Information Source
www.crinfo.org

Conflict Resolution Model Texas Board of Nurse Examiners
http://www.bne.state.tx.us/conflict.htm

Journal of Conflict Resolution
http://www.jstor.org/journals/00220027.html

Surviving Conflict on the Job
http://nsweb.nursingspectrum.com/cfforms/GuestLecture/survivingconflict.cfm

CHAPTER

11

TEAM BUILDING SKILLS

committee
dysfunctional team roles
functional team roles
group
group meetings

interdisciplinary
task force
team
team-building tools
team development process

INTRODUCTION

Teams are more than just groups—they are people who come together to fulfill a specific purpose. Teams may be ongoing, or they may be formed for a specific, time-limited objective. All teams seem to go through predictable stages or development. In addition, all teams must deal with members who do and do not function well. Nurse leaders who lead teams use a variety of skills to facilitate teams so that they function to the best of their ability.

KEY POINTS

1. Definition. A **team** is a "small number of people with complementary skills who are committed to a common purpose, performance goals, and approach for which they hold themselves accountable" (Katzenbach & Smith, 1993, p. 45). A team is more purposeful than a **group**, which is an aggregate of individuals who interact and mutually influence each other (Shaw, 1981).

   A. Teams are both more and less efficient than individuals.

      i. more efficient

        a. more resources, ideas, abilities

        b. able to see a larger variety of perspectives and possibilities

   ii. less efficient

        a. more potential for conflict

        b. requires more time to accomplish many tasks

B.   Different types of teams. Teams can follow a number of configurations. Two key types are:

    i. **interdisciplinary** teams

        a. composed of members with a variety of clinical expertise, for example, nurses, physicians, respiratory and physical therapists, social workers, case managers, etc

        b. work best when everyone is heard and able to contribute his or her expertise

        c. team leader's role is to ensure that all team members have a chance to participate and contribute, particularly focusing on their areas of expertise

        d. this type of team is often permanent or ongoing

   ii. **committee** or **task force**

        a. team that is brought together to accomplish a specific task or goal, for example, an ad hoc committee to study the feasibility of a mobile mammography center

        b. in some cases, standing committees may meet on a long-term, regular schedule; for example, a standing committee on ethics or accrediting standards

        c. committees can recommend action, take action, or serve in an advisory role (Polifko-Harris, 2003)

  iii. groups that are not teams

        a. informal groups (usually social, not defined by organizational structure), such as people who are interested in a particular hobby or activity

        b. competing groups (members compete for resources or recognition)

        c. ordinary interacting groups (members interact and may influence one another but do not have a collective purpose) (Sullivan & Decker, 2001)

C.   How teams work. Most groups have predictable phases of development and functioning.

    i. **team development process** consists of the following five steps

        a. forming: The initial stage of group development; individuals assemble into a well-defined team. For example, three RNs, two social workers, a physician, a respiratory therapist, a case manager, and a hospital chaplain form an ethics committee that examines how a hospital deals with critically ill trauma patients and their families.

b. storming: Members develop roles and relationships; some competition and conflict may occur. For example, in this development stage, the ethics team would define how team members function (advisory, policy making) and would decide which members have formal leadership roles; in this case, the physician may assume the leader's role by virtue of title, when that role may not be appropriate at all.

c. norming: Members define their goals and rules of behavior. For example, for an ethics committee, members might decide the kinds of cases they will examine, and may agree on an ethical philosophy or guide to follow.

d. performing: Members agree on basic activities and carry out the committee's stated work. For example, the ethics committee would meet on the second Tuesday of each month from 3:00 to 5:30 p.m., and could listen to a case study about an ethically challenging case (such as an 18-year old who said he would rather be dead than paralyzed and refused emergency care in the trauma room of the ER) or to deal with issues raised by patients or staff.

e. adjourning: The team dissolves after achieving its objectives (unless it becomes a permanent committee).

f. re-forming: The team reassembles after a major change in the hospital environment or after the team's goals or activities change significantly. For example, the team re-forms after agreeing to focus only on issues concerning hospice care (Sullivan & Decker, 2001).

D. Roles of group members

i. all groups have both functional and dysfunctional members; people may or may not be aware of the role(s) they are playing

ii. **functional roles** for team members include:

a. creator: the person who gets the ball rolling, supplies ideas and initiative

b. coordinator: the person who is able to see the project as a whole and can bring together a variety of resources to keep the project moving forward

c. mobilizer: the person who keeps other team members energized and moving forward; helps provide the spark, especially in difficult or challenging times

d. recorder: the person who keeps track of the details, including team meeting details, schedules, and progress (Polifko-Harris, 2003)

e. information giver/seeker: the person who asks questions to gauge the team's knowledge, or who gives the group relevant information

f. tension-breaker: the person who uses humor, listening, or other skills to relieve the team's tension and refocus it on its task (Locker, 1995)

g. note that each of these roles can be assumed by a nurse leader, as leaders accomplish goals in many and varied ways

iii. **dysfunctional roles** for team members include:

a. criticizers or naysayers: respond negatively to any team action without offering alternatives or constructive advice

b. passives: refuse to take a stand; often indecisive and reluctant to provide any kind of input

c. detailers: lose the big picture in the details; often get side-tracked (and try to sidetrack others) (Polifko-Harris, 2003)

d. dominators: "take over" every meeting, insisting that they talk the most, and not letting others participate

e. clowns: people who use humor inappropriately to distract the group from its purpose (Locker, 1995)

iv. behaviors needed for groups to function effectively

a. have a clearly stated purpose: goals, objectives, how long and how often the team will meet, vision, and balance of larger goals of organization and smaller goals of team

b. assess the team's composition: team members' strengths and weaknesses; interactive dynamics between team members; how team perceives itself (as individuals or as team); keeping in mind that individuals are more important than job titles; for example, not every social worker would be an effective team member as different social workers bring different strengths to the table; some are experts at coordinating resources for discharge planning, while others are experts in counseling

c. use effective communication strategies: both written and verbal communication tools or technology that the team needs to stay connected and informed; communication style of team members (both listening and speaking skills)

d. all members actively participate in the team's work: each team member has a designated responsibility; leader must resolve any turf issues at the start.

e. have a clear plan for proceeding: everyone needs to agree on the plan; it should be revisited periodically and members need to provide regular feedback (both top to bottom and bottom to top) about the plan

f. continuously evaluate and assess the team and its work

2. **Team-building tools.** A number of team enhancement tools are available for leaders to use. These tools generally help team members assess characteristics such as personality or work style. The idea is that if team members understand how they work, they will be more able to recognize elements that can cause team conflict and develop ways to decrease conflict and increase team effectiveness. Some frequently used tools are briefly described as follows:

A.   DISC Behavioral Model

   i.   assesses behaviors that people use in groups
   ii. behaviors are categorized as follows:
      a. dominant: a high "D" person is a leader; likes to be in charge and direct others; he or she is task-oriented, has a strong ego, and enjoys challenges; this person may be impatient and is not always trusting
      b. interactive: a high "I" person likes people and tends to be optimistic and people-oriented; this person dislikes social rejection and disorganization
      c. steady: a high "S" person likes to serve others, and is usually a very good team player; this person tends to be loyal and likes to see concrete results; he or she can become possessive if feeling insecure or overextended
      d. compliant: a high "C" person has very high internal standards and works hard to meet them; this person has a strong need for accuracy and may be critical of the work of himself/herself and others (Target Training International, 1994)

B.   Hermann Brain Dominance Model

   i.   emphasizes the four quadrants of brain function (A, B, C, and D), each of which has its own language, values, and behavior. Quadrants A and D are considered "cerebral" elements while B and C are "limbic" elements.
   ii. generally a person shows a preference (dominance) for using two or three quadrants
      a. quadrant A: looking for data, analyzing, critical thinking
      b. quadrant B: detail work, finding practical applications, using methodical learning strategies
      c. quadrant C: sharing ideas and intuition, group work, less interested in details
      d. quadrant D: big picture, problem solving, exploring long-range goals

C.   Myers-Briggs type indicator (MBTI)

   i.   based on a person's preferred modes of interacting with people and information

    ii. categories include
- a. extrovert/introvert (whether a person is energized by people or ideas)
- b. intuitive/sensing (whether a person processes information primarily through intuition or the five senses)
- c. thinking/feeling (whether a person decides based on logic or emotion)
- d. judging/perceiving (whether a person prefers a more methodical or spontaneous approach to tasks) (Kiersey & Bates, 1989)

D.   Gregorc Style Delineator

    i. focuses on "mind mediation channels" that identify how people best process incoming information

    ii. two characteristics are
- a. nature of content, abstract (world of ideas) or concrete (world that must be validated by the five senses)
- b. ordering of content, random (no particular order, haphazard) or sequential (a logical, predictable order)

    iii. these characteristics are combined into four channels
- a. concrete sequential: this person sees the world as objective and predictable; uses methodical and deliberate thinking processes; prefers a stable environment; and tends to learn best hands on, doing something step by step
- b. abstract sequential: this person sees the world as having metaphysical aspects; uses logical, intellectual thinking processes; and prefers a stable environment with few distractions
- c. abstract random: this person sees the world as social, with feelings and emotions; uses feelings as a key part of the thinking process; and prefers a busy environment with a lot of social interaction
- d. concrete random: this person sees the world in terms of intuition and instinct; uses quick, impulsive thinking processes, and thrives on a stimulating, change-filled environment (Carroll, 1992)

    iv. nurse leaders who know how their staff members and colleagues see the world, think, and deal with interactions with others can, for example, place two people with similar mediation channels to work together on a unit, while ensuring that a mix of mediation channels are present on a team that will set policy for the entire organization.

3. The leader as **facilitator.** The word "facilitate" is based on "facile" or easy. Thus, a facilitator tries to make something less difficult or remove impediments from the process. Being a group facilitator is a key skill for nurse leaders. The leader must balance a number of often competing agendas (personal, organizational, group dynamics, resources) in order to help the group function easily and efficiently.

A. Qualities of an effective facilitator. According to Costello-Nickitas (1997), an effective team facilitator:

    i.   is sensitive to the needs and emotions of the group

    ii. can gauge the group's energy level and is aware of its stress levels

    iii. can be a role model while also enabling groups to share responsibility and use their skills to accomplish goals

B. Responsibilities of a facilitator. An effective facilitator is responsible for:

    i.   guiding without directing (helping team members find solutions, but not telling them what the solution "should be")

    ii. making changes without disruption (for example, bringing a new resource to the attention of team members, and then letting them decide when and how to use it)

    iii. helping team members discover new approaches and solutions (by providing feedback, resources, networks to other teams, etc.) as well as by motivating and encouraging team members to continue toward their goal

    iv. appreciating and using diversity (more diverse teams may experience more conflict but they also have significantly more potential resources than do nondiverse teams)

C. Promoting full group participation. An effective facilitator makes sure that all team members feel confident and safe to contribute their ideas. To do this, the facilitator must create a climate of participation, generally by using the following types of questions:

    i.   direct question that requires a direct response from a team member, for example, "Sam, what do you think about the new workflow that we're considering?"

    ii. general question that allows anyone on the team to respond, for example, "Who has insights on the best way to coordinate the upcoming visit from the JCAHO team?"

    iii. return question that asks a team member to elaborate further; for example, "Bobby, you asked how we can lower the number of medication errors on the CCU; where do you think we need to start?"

    iv. relay question that includes people who have not yet joined in the discussion; for example, "Nic, you've worked with the 'cell phone on call' system for about a year now. Could you summarize for us what has been successful in that program?"

D.   Dealing with diversity. To deal with diversity, an effective facilitator:

  i.   addresses different ideas and perspectives so that the team mem-
       bers better understand the issues and their implications
  ii. allows different ideas to emerge and be heard so that the group
       has many possible alternatives to choose from
  iii. makes sure every team member's ideas and thoughts are heard
  iv. generates energy and moves the team toward resolution of the
       issue, problem, or task

4. Conducting effective **group meetings.** A key skill for facilitating teams
   effectively is being able to conduct effective meetings. Meetings in most
   organizations are notorious for being poorly run time wasters. According
   to Costello-Nickitas (1997), the following steps will allow nurse leaders
   and facilitators to conduct effective team meetings

A   Preparation

  i.   decide if the meeting is really necessary
       a. is a face-to-face discussion necessary?
       b. could the same or more be accomplished through informal
          conversations or other communication strategies?
  ii. define the meeting's purpose and desired outcome; meetings are
       generally needed when
       a. information is scattered among different team members and
          needs to be communicated to all members
       b. team members need to agree on a key point before moving
          forward
       c. there is a lack of structure or focus about the problem or issue
       d. people have competing agendas, and a face-to-face meeting
          lets everyone hear the same information at the same time,
          with the benefit of tone of voice and body language
  iii. decide who needs to attend the meeting
  iv. evaluate the chemistry of the team members, including
       a. power and influence
       b. interest and enthusiasm
       c. general demeanor (open, skeptical, hostile)
  v.   set the specific meeting agenda
       a. person calling the meeting
       b. people invited to the meeting
       c. date, start time, and end time
       d. meeting place
       e. meeting purpose (and action items, if needed)

B.   Managing meeting dynamics

  i.   unite the group

    a. promote harmony within the team and help balance members' energy and emotions

    b. allow anger and frustration to be expressed appropriately and worked through

    c. stick to the facts of any conflict

    d. avoid taking sides in any conflict

  ii. focus the group

    a. keep the group on track, especially if attention starts to wander in mid-meeting

    b. test for understanding

    c. use active listening, paraphrasing, summarizing and other techniques to keep group on task

  iii. mobilize the group

    a. encourage all team members to participate

    b. help team members work toward consensus

    c. record any outcomes

    d. set time and essential tasks for next meeting, if needed

REVIEW ACTIVITIES

Questions

1. The key difference between a team and a group is:

  a. the number of members

  b. the level of formality

  c. whether they have a specific goal

  d. the length of time when it is active

2. Which of the following is true about an interdisciplinary team?

  a. it is composed of members from one organizational area only

  b. it works best when everyone is heard and is able to contribute his or her expertise

  c. team leader's role is to ensure that team members do not spend too much time at meetings

  d. it is seldom an ongoing entity

3. In this stage of the team development process, members define their goals and rules of behavior:

  a. norming

  b. storming

  c. performing

  d. re-forming

4. Some conflict or competition may occur in this stage of team development.
   a. norming
   b. storming
   c. performing
   d. forming

5. This negative team behavior, which involves not letting other team members participate, is called:
   a. dominating
   b. clowning
   c. detailing
   d. information giving

6. A team member who uses humor, listening, or other skills to decrease conflict and refocus the team on its task is called a(n):
   a. dominator
   b. criticizer
   c. information seeker
   d. tension breaker

7. This team-building tool assesses behaviors that people use in groups:
   a. Myers-Briggs type indicator
   b. DISC model
   c. Hermann Brain Dominance Model
   d. Gregorc Style Delineator

8. An effective facilitator manages team dynamics by:
   a. taking sides to settle conflicts
   b. allowing the group to indirectly reach its purpose or objective
   c. encourage the group to stay on task and continue toward its objectives
   d. excluding difficult people from the group

Critical Thinking Questions

1. List appropriate team members by job title (such as nurse, social worker, respiratory therapist) to form teams to tackle these issues:
   a. working with people with terminal illness to determine what treatments they want and which they do not
   b. developing a school-based asthma management program
   c. developing a care path for patients undergoing lower extremity joint replacement surgery
   d. establishing a community health care center for the medically underserved

e. assuring continuity of care for patients whose stroke treatment begins in the acute care hospital ED and continues, using a variety of community resources

f. enhancing efficiency in the operating rooms so that there is minimal downtime between procedures

Discussion Questions

1. Which teams do you belong to in your school or workplace? How do they function? What is their task? Is there any way by which they could function more effectively?

2. Choose a team leader you know and evaluate his or her facilitation skills. Based on your experience, what makes a leader an effective facilitator?

Works Cited

Carroll, P. (1992). Using personality styles to enhance preceptor programs. *Dimensions of Critical Care Nursing, 11*(2), 114–121.

Costello-Nickitas, D. (1997). *Quick reference to nursing leadership.* Clifton Park, NY: Thomson Delmar Learning.

Katzenbach, J. R., & Smith, D. K. (1993). *The wisdom of teams: Creating the high-performance organization.* New York: Harper Business.

Kiersey, D., & Bates, M. (1989). *Please Understand Me, An Essay on Temperament Styles.* Del Mar, CA: Prometheus Nemesis Books.

Locker, K. O. (1995). *Business and administrative communication* (3rd ed). Chicago: Irwin.

Polifko-Harris, K. (2003). Effective team building. In P. Kelly-Heidenthal (Ed.), *Nursing leadership & management* (pp. 202–216). Clifton Park, NY: Thomson Delmar Learning.

Shaw, M. E. (1981). *Group dynamics* (3rd ed). New York: McGraw-Hill.

Sullivan, E. J., & Decker, P. J. (2001). *Effective leadership and management in nursing,* (5th ed.). Upper Saddle River, N.J.: Prentice Hall.

Target Training International. (1994). Managing for Success: DISC. Employee-Manager Packet.

Additional Resources

Bell, M. (2002). A virtual team group process. *Canadian Journal of Nursing Leadership, 15*(3), 30–33.

Emmet, C. E. (2003). Team building is the key to promote professionalism. Hospital changes are no excuse for bad behavior (Management help line, April). *RN, 66*(9), 10, 13.

Fitzgerald, A. (2004). Health reform, professional identity and occupational subcultures: The changing interprofessional relations between doctors and nurses. *Contemporary Nurse, 16*(1–2), 9–19.

Hill, K. S. (2003). Development of leadership competencies as a team. *Journal of Nursing Administration, 33*(12), 639–642.

Hoban, B. (2003). Careers. How to manage a meeting. *Nursing Times, 99*(21), 64–65.

Horak, B. J. (2004). Patient safety: A case study in team building and interdisciplinary collaboration. *Journal of Healthcare Quality, 26*(2), 6–13, 60.

Laing, K. (2003). Teambuilding. *Gastroenterology Nurse, 26*(4), 156–158.

McWilliam, C. L. et al. (2003). Building empowering partnerships for interprofessional care. *Journal of Interprofessional Care, 17*(4), 363–377.

Oliver, D. (2003). Use of a pro forma and overhead projector to improve multidisciplinary team communication. *International Journal of Palliative Nursing, 9*(8), 358–359.

Web Sites

Online DISC Profile Kit
http://www.onlinediscprofile.com

Gregorc Associates: Gregorc Style Delineator
http://www.gregorc.com

Team Building Activities
http://www.teamdevelopment.com/tryathome.htm

Team Building for Patient Safety: National Association for Healthcare Quality
http://www.nahq.org/journal/ce/article.html?article_id=171

Team Building Games and Exercises
http://www.businessballs.com/businessballs.htm

Part III

Putting the Primary Skills to Work: Strategic Organizational Roles for the Nursing Leader

CHAPTER

12

MANAGING FIRST-LINE PATIENT CARE

accountability-based care

competency

goals

hospital information systems

management information systems

mission statement

nursing information systems

objectives

patient care management

patient-focused care

shared governance

situational leadership

strategic planning

SWOT analysis

vision statement

INTRODUCTION

The nurse leader in first-line patient care management fills a crucial role in planning, implementing, and evaluating patient care outcomes. This complex role requires flexible leadership skills, the ability to see both short-term and long-term goals, and the ability to design and implement strategic plans. A nurse leader in this role in an organization may very well be a key participant in various councils, committees, or workgroups that oversee different aspects of patient care management. In addition, being effective in this role requires familiarity with automation and management information systems.

1. Definition

    A. First-line **patient care management** uses nursing process to plan, implement, and evaluate care outcomes for patient populations (rather than for individual patients). Effective first-line patient care management requires:

        i. a manager who leads and coordinates a team of diverse individuals toward a common goal (MacGregor-Burns, 1979)

     ii. governance structures, patient care delivery processes, and measures of care delivery outcomes, all of which are consistent with professional practice philosophy and the organization's vision

     iii. shared decision making between nursing leaders and nursing staff

     iv. environment in which patient care delivery, clinical quality, access, service, and cost are accountable and can be evaluated (Sellers, 2003)

  B. Leadership skills are essential in managing first-line patient care

     i. manager/leader directs a complex team with varied skills and knowledge; for example, the nurse leader responsible for first-line patient care management may direct staff ranging from non-credentialed technicians to RNs to physicians to social workers to clergy

     ii. the goal is to achieve best patient care outcomes

2. Strategic planning is a process designed to achieve goals in dynamic environments through allocating resources (Andrews, 1990). This type of planning is essential to managing first-line patient care.

  A. Components of strategic planning include:

     i. assessing internal and external environments, such as staffing levels, age of workforce (internal) and competition from other organizations or changes in government and other third party reimbursement schedules (external)

       a. conducting environmental assessments of existing possibilities and risks

       b. may be in the form of a **SWOT** (Strengths, Weaknesses, Opportunities, and Threats) **analysis**

     ii. developing a philosophy or belief statement that reflects an organization's core values. These statements can include:

       a. **mission statement:** a brief, fairly broad statement that reflects the organization's purpose, its key principles or values, and its customers or clients

       b. **vision statement:** a statement that reflects the organization's work, why and how it is done, thus anchoring the vision to reality (Wesorick et al., 1997)

       c. statements of **goals** (specific target to achieve) or **objectives** (measurable steps taken to reach a goal): strategies that span three to five years, and specify annual actions needed to attain the goals

     iii. professional practice structure

       a. **shared governance** frameworks: an organizational framework based on the concept of decentralized leadership and

autonomous decision making (Porter-O'Grady, 1992). In this structure, nursing leadership would be responsible for dealing with the overall organizational structure and resources, while leaving clinical decisions on the unit to the nurses on staff.
  b. clinical practice council: establishes practice standard for work groups using evidence-based practice plus research initiatives
  c. quality council: designed to set standards for staff, interview and hire candidates that meet specified criteria. They also oversee a unit's quality management initiatives, including whether to retain, promote, or terminate the staff, based on established indicators.
  d. education council: assesses staff education/learning needs and develops and implements programs to meet these needs. A hospital's education council may provide educational opportunities ranging from new employee orientation, to continuing clinical education, to training all staff to use new equipment or management information systems.
  e. research council: advances research, with the goal of incorporating results into evidence-based clinical practice; this council may also coordinate research projects conducted at the institution
  f. management council: ensures that practice and governance standards agreed on by the staff are upheld and that there are sufficient resources available to deliver those standards. A first-line patient care manager is always a standing member of this council.
  g. coordinating council: facilitates and integrates the activities of all the other councils (often made up of the first-line patient care manager plus chairpersons from all the other councils). This council may also facilitate annual reviews of mission and vision and develop the annual operational plan (Sellers, 1996).
  iv. ensuring staff competency and continued development
  a. **competency** means possessing the required skill(s), knowledge, qualification or capacity and performing with these skills in the clinical setting; this quality is best determined in practice by a group of peers; competency is not properly assessed by written examinations
  b. competency and development of professional staff are ensured through credentialing processes and continuing education, or by the person being promoted to higher levels in an organization because of clinical performance

B. Developing expertise

  i. **situational leadership**, according to Hersey and Blanchard (1993), has these characteristics:
  a. there is no one "best" leadership style, but effective leadership lies in matching a leader's style to staff's level of readiness

(ability and motivation to perform a task) and the circumstances under which the leader must act

   b. as staff grows in its level of ability, situational leader adopts leadership style to match new level of staff expertise or ability

   c. the higher the staff's readiness and expertise, the less control the situational leader needs to exert; this is a key aspect for nurse leader to understand as highly skilled staff's morale and performance can be harmed by too much control from the management

   d. developing staff based on their readiness levels facilitates their movement from "beginner to expert" (Benner, 1984) and ensures a care team that is consistently and accountably able to deliver appropriate patient care

C.   Method of first-line patient care delivery

   i. **accountability-based care** delivery

     a. accountable means being able to report, explain, or justify one's actions

     b. accountability-based care delivery systems assume that the system is accountable to the patients who receive nursing care. In primary nursing care, for example, one nurse is accountable for a patient's care during the entire episode of care, from admission to discharge and 24 hours a day. Because of primary nursing's dependence on the use of registered nurses (which requires higher budgets than a mixed staff), many delivery systems are not able to support this method; the current shortage of qualified registered nurses also makes this model difficult to implement in today's health care environment.

   ii. **patient-focused care**

     a. emphasizes quality, cost, and value (Reisdorfer, 1996)

     b. first-line patient care manager has an expanded role that includes coordinating and overseeing all care activities, including managing nurses and staff from a variety of departments such as radiology or physical therapy

     c. relies more on a mixed staff containing assistive workers trained by the organization without external standards of practice

     d. some have suggested that the name "patient-focused" care is a smokescreen that sounds as if the model is in the patient's interest, but actually hides the reduction of registered nurse staff

   iii. **case management**

     a. this accountability-based system evolved in the late 1980s and early 1990s as a result of skyrocketing health care costs

b. primary goal is to deliver high-quality patient care in the most cost-effective way by managing human and material resources

c. other goals include managing care within a given timeframe, decreasing length of inpatient care, ensuring continuity of care, and standardizing care for a given diagnosis (Sellers, 2003)

D. Determining measurable outcomes

    i. key component of first-line patient care management is to regularly evaluate performance to ensure that care outcomes meet established objectives

    ii. process improvement measurements in current organizations are driven by

        a. Joint Commission on Accreditation of Healthcare Organizations (JCAHO)

        b. National Council for Quality Assurance (NCQA)

        c. governmental agencies such as the Center for Medicare and Medicaid Services and state regulations

    iii. unit-based quality improvement to meet accountability requirements needs to track four outcome domains: access, service, costs, and clinical quality

    iv. one source of outcomes data in the managed care industry is the Quality Compass from the National Committee for Quality Assurance (NCQA), which measures quality of functional status, clinical outcomes, cost/utilization, and patient satisfaction for managed care organizations (Sellers, 2003)

3. The role of **management information systems** in patient care management. According to Sullivan and Decker, management information systems are key to an organization's ability to collect, use, and store information, which in turn is key to effectively managing patient care.

A. Types of information systems

    i. **management information systems**

        a. capture data about an organization's services, employees, and patients

        b. can include analytical tools, operating policies, and communication protocols that support management decisions

    ii. **hospital information systems**

        a. integrated system to manage patient information

        b. tracks patient appointments, admissions, transfers, discharges, medication orders and profiles, critical pathways, and patient acuities

        c. information may be part of a network that extends beyond the hospital to include physicians, pharmacies, and laboratories

    d. when ideally designed, these systems protect patient privacy while enhancing continuity of care and rapid access to key patient data

    e. the best information systems allow managers to pose questions and get answers from the database such as, "how many patients were seen in the ER during shifts on which nurses worked overtime?"

  iii. **nursing information systems**

    a. integrated system to manage patient information

    b. includes care plans, charting, and orders

    c. systems are becoming more complex and increasingly include patient records, outcome data, and acuity calculations

  iv. nursing information system applications

    a. patient care module used to assess patient acuity, prepare appropriate care plan or critical path, plan specific interventions, document care, and track outcomes. An increasing number of these tools are moving to the wireless and/or handheld technology domain (McGrow, Roys, Maloney, & Xiao, 2004; Tooey & Mayo, 2004).

    b. provide ready reference tools for clinical practice such as drug guides, formula calculators, procedures and protocols and others appropriate to a specific practice setting (ED, critical care, perioperative, pediatrics, etc.), and on-demand clinical education programs

    c. patient monitoring systems can provide measurements (such as IV administration), and surveillance (such as pulse oximetry)

    d. patient management systems assist nurses with decision making and monitoring, such as electrocardiographic monitoring that calculates ST-segment elevation and identifies changes consistent with myocardial ischemia and those that provide special alerts when life-threatening dysrhythmias are detected

    e. nursing management systems can provide fiscal management, employee data, scheduling, and quality improvement and utilization review

    f. communication systems allow linked computers to share information seamlessly; these can include local area networks (LAN), wide area networks (WAN), wireless networks, the Internet, and telehealth applications

    g. other applications include using computer-based distance learning for continuing education, as well as research

B. Advantages of using information systems

  i. automated systems link departments and allow sharing of large amounts of data and allow decisions to be based on hard data

  ii. increased access to information

       iii. lower costs by saving time

       iv. improved employee retention and satisfaction (through automating "paperwork" and providing more patient contact time)

  C. Disadvantages of using information systems

       i. resistance by users who are computer phobic or who see automation as loss of control over patient care

       ii. cost for initial set up

       iii. potential for compromise of security

       iv. system down time

  D. All systems must now meet the requirements of the Health Insurance Portability and Accountability Act that sets out specific requirements for sharing patient information (see Web sites for additional information).

REVIEW ACTIVITIES

Questions

1. Which of the following is true about patient care management?

  a. it uses medical process to plan, implement, and evaluate care outcomes

  b. it focuses on patient populations rather than individual patients

  c. it links computers to share information seamlessly

  d. it achieves goals in dynamic environments through allocating resources

2. A mission statement is best defined as:

  a. a brief, fairly broad statement that reflects the organization's purpose, its key principles or values, and its customers or clients

  b. a statement that reflects the organization's work, why and how it is done

  c. annual actions specified as needed to attain the goals

  d. an organizational framework of decentralized leadership and autonomous decision making

3. A council that establishes practice standards for work groups using evidence-based practice is called:

  a. a quality council

  b. a management council

  c. an education council

  d. a research council

4. Which of the following statements about competency is correct?
   a. it means possessing the required skills, knowledge, qualification or capacity
   b. it cannot be determined by peers and must be determined by supervisors
   c. it is best evaluated by credentialing or continuing education
   d. it is not a requirement for promotion in an organization

5. Which of the following systems evolved in response to rising health care costs?
   a. situational leadership
   b. shared governance
   c. case management
   d. JCAHO

6. These information systems collect data about an organization's services, employees, and patients, and can include analytical tools, operating policies, and communication protocols.
   a. management information systems
   b. hospital information systems
   c. nursing information systems
   d. telehealth information systems

7. These systems are used to assess patient acuity, prepare appropriate care plan or critical path, specific interventions, document care, and track outcomes.
   a. management information systems
   b. hospital information systems
   c. nursing information systems
   d. telehealth information systems

Critical Thinking Questions

1. A 150-bed community hospital has decided to implement an automated order-entry system that will require all orders for patient care to be entered electronically. Users who are authorized to write orders can access the system from any computer with access to the network. Develop a plan for implementing this system. Include three benefits of such a system that should be emphasized as well as three potential barriers that must be overcome.

2. Does your nursing school have a mission and vision statement? If yes, analyze it with regard to current challenges facing nursing education. If no, write a mission and vision statement for the program.

Discussion Questions

1. In the health care organization (or nursing unit) with which you are most familiar, who is the person (or people) responsible for first-line patient care management? What leadership qualities do you observe in this person?

2. Find the mission and vision statements for the health care organization in which you most recently had a clinical experience. How well does it meet the criteria for these statements discussed in this chapter? How do the mission and vision statements compare with your personal experiences in this organization?

3. Choose a health care organization in which you have worked as a staff or in which you have spent time as a student. What care delivery system does the organization follow? What are its strengths and weaknesses?

4. Analyze a health care organization with which you are familiar and note the information systems in place. How many systems and tasks are automated? How do these systems make your work more or less productive? Are the systems seamlessly integrated throughout the organization, or are different systems used in different departments?

Works Cited

Andrews, J. (1984). Designing a competency-based orientation for critical care nurses. *Heart and Lung, 13*, 655–662.

Benner, P. (1984). *From novice to expert*. Menlo Park, CA: Addison-Wesley Publishing.

Hersey, R. E., & Blanchard, T. (1993). *Management of organizational behavior*. Edgewood Cliffs, NJ: Prentice-Hall.

MacGregor-Burns, J. (1979). *Leadership*. New York: Harper & Row.

McGraw, K. M., Roys, R., Maloney, R. C., & Xiao, Y. (2004). Informatics: Using wireless technologies to improve information flow for interhospital transfers of critical care patients. *Critical Care Nurse, 24*(2), 66–72.

Porter-O'Grady, T. (1992). *Implementing shared governance: Creating a professional organization*. St. Louis, MO: Mosby Year Book.

Reisdorfer, J. T. (1996). Building a patient-focused care unit. *Nursing Management, 27*(10), 38, 40, 42, 44.

Sellers, K. F. (1996). *The meaning of autonomous nursing practice to staff nurses in a shared governance organization: A hermeneutical analysis*. Unpublished doctoral dissertation, Adelphi University, Garden City, New York.

Sellers, K. F. (2003). First-line patient care management. In P. Kelly-Heidenthal (Ed.), *Nursing leadership & management* (pp. 280–299). Clifton Park, NY: Thomson Delmar Learning.

Sullivan, E. J., & Decker, P. J. (2001). *Effective leadership and management in nursing* (5th ed.). Upper Saddle River, NJ.: Prentice Hall.

Tooey, M. J., & Mayo, A. (2004). Handheld technologies in a clinical setting: State of the technology and resources. *Critical Care Nurse*, 24(1), 28–30, 32, 34–38.

Wesorick, B., Shiparski, L., Bott, M., & Taunton, R. L. (1995, December). Shared governance: From vision to reality. *Journal of Nursing Administration*, 25(12), 45–54.

Additional Resources

American Nurses Association. (1999). *Competencies for telehealth technologies in nursing.* Washington, D.C.: Author.

American Nurses Association. (2002). *Clinical information systems: A framework for reaching the vision.* (includes "Scope and standards of nursing informatics practice"). Washington, D.C: Author.

Contino, D. S. (2004). Leadership competencies: Knowledge, skills, and aptitudes nurses need to lead organizations effectively. *Critical Care Nurse*, 24(3), 52–58, 60–64.

Currell, R., & Urquhart, C. (2004). Nursing records systems: Effects on nursing practice and health care outcomes. The Cochrane Library. Available at: http://www.update-software.com/Abstracts/AB002099.htm.

Hess, R. (January 31, 2004) "From Bedside to Boardroom—Nursing Shared Governance."*Online Journal of Issues in Nursing*, 9(1). Available at: www.nursingworld.org/ojin/topic23/tpc23_1.htm.

Laughlin, J., & Van Null, M. (2003). Boost regulatory compliance with electronic nursing documentation. *Nursing Management*, 34(12), 51–52.

O'Neill, E. S., Dluhy, N. M., Fortier, P. J., & Michel, H. E. (2004). Knowledge acquisition, synthesis, and validation: A model for decision support systems. *Journal of Advanced Nursing*, 47(2), 134–143.

Roark, D. C. (2004). Bar codes and drug administration: Can new technology reduce the number of medication errors? *American Journal of Nursing*, 104(1), 63–66.

Smith, C. (2004). New technology continues to invade health care: What are the strategic implications/outcomes? *Nursing Administration Quarterly*, 28(2), 92–99.

Web Sites

American Health Information Management Association
http://www.ahima.org/

American Medical Informatics Association
http://www.amia.org

American Nursing Informatics Association
http://www.ania.org

Health Insurance Portability and Accountability Act Resources from the U.S. Department of Health and Human Services
http://www.hhs.gov/ocr/hipaa/

Joint Commission on Accreditation of Healthcare Organizations (JCAHO)
http://www.jcaho.org

New Healthcare Delivery System
http://www.afscme.org/una/nurse07.htm

Nursing Shared Governance
http://www.harthosp.org/nursing/workplace/governance.html

http://www.seton.net/Employment7/Nursing/SharedGovernance.asp

Online Journal of Nursing Informatics
http://www.nursing-informatics.com

SWOT Analysis
http://www.mindtools.com/swot.html

What's in a Vision Statement?
http://www.allianceonline.org/FAQ/strategic_planning/what_s_in_vision_statement.faq

Writing a Mission Statement
http://www.bplans.com/dp/missionstatement.cfm

CHAPTER
13

STRATEGIC THINKING TO IMPROVE PATIENT CARE (INCLUDING EVIDENCE-BASED CARE)

INTRODUCTION

Evidence-based care uses the best current research and data to make the most effective decisions about patient care. Planning, implementing, evaluating, and documenting care that is based on this information has become a key component of nursing, and this trend will continue.

Nurse leaders must not only evaluate the available research to guide care planning, they also have to coordinate interdisciplinary teams carrying out and documenting evidence-based care. This chapter defines evidence-based care, emphasizes its importance, provides examples of current models being used in health care, and outlines basis steps for moving from theory to practice in health care organizations.

KEY POINTS

1. What is **evidence-based care**?

   A. Definition

      i. the "conscientious, explicit, and judicious use of current best evidence in making decisions about the care of individual patients" (Sackett, et al., 1996) (also called evidence-based practice)

    ii. uses outcomes research and other current research findings to
       guide the development of appropriate strategies to deliver qual-
       ity and cost-effective care
       a. **Outcomes research** determines what actions and conditions
          produce which outcomes or results
    iii. looks to outcomes research evidence for treatment benefits, risks,
       and results so that people can make informed decisions about
       care (Jadlos, 2003)

B. Evidence-based practice competencies. The Pew Health Professions
    Commission (Bellack & O'Neill, 2000) identified a number of **evidence-
    based practice competencies** that 21st century health care professionals
    would need for the practice environments and health care organizations
    of the future. The four key competencies related to outcomes are:

    i. provide evidence-based, clinically competent care
    ii. demonstrate critical thinking, reflection, and problem-solving skills
    iii. take responsibility for care quality and health outcomes at all levels
    iv. contribute to continuous improvement of the health care system

C. How evidence-based practice has developed

    i. historical development
       a. historically, health care relied on biomedical parameters or
          diagnostic tests to determine whether a health intervention is
          needed and nursing practice, in particular, has historically
          been based on interventions provided because "we've always
          done it this way"
       b. health care professionals realized that these biomedical tests
          measure only a fraction of the multidimensional outcomes
          that matter to patients (for example quality of life, overall
          level of functioning)
       c. some patient satisfaction data (for example, using surveys)
          has been collected, but historically these surveys did not
          address the range of patient criteria (Clancy & Eisenberg,
          1998; Jadlos, 2003)
    ii. current definitions and nurses' roles
       a. **evidence-based nursing practice** is the "conscientious,
          explicit, and judicious use of theory-derived, research-based
          information in making decisions about nursing care delivery
          to individuals or groups of individuals and in consideration of
          individual needs and preferences" (Ingersoll, 2000)
       b. nurses' role is to participate in developing a comprehensive,
          interdisciplinary plan of care that integrates the art and science
          of caring, not merely the medical model of the absence or pres-
          ence of disease (Jadlos, 2003)

      c. nurses should also be innovative and creative and use technology to move beyond the traditional mindset that focused on what nurses do instead of integrating what nurses know with what nurses do (Bryant, 1998, cited in Jadlos, 2003)

      d. professional organizations such as the American Nurses Association (ANA) are actively involved in setting standards for evidence-based nursing practice

E.   Why is evidence-based care important?

     i. patients, health care providers, and payers recognize the significance of collecting data and analyzing outcomes to achieve optimum care

    ii. outcome strategies developed in evidence-based practice are based on science, not tradition, and used to create clinical protocols, guidelines, pathways, and algorithms, which are the key tools for health care interventions

   iii. evidence-based practice is most successful when the entire organization is invested in the process and participates in and supports it

   iv. evidence-based practice has become the key to identifying and developing better strategies to monitor and improve quality of care (Jadlos, 2003)

2. Developing and evaluating evidence: nursing evidence reports. The volume and variety of **nursing research** being done can make it difficult for nurses to decide which evidence is more reliable and which can be used as a basis for evidence-based practice. According to Stetler et al., (1998), most research falls into the following six categories (listed from most to least reliable).

A.   meta-analysis of multiple controlled studies

     i. findings from several randomized, controlled research studies on a topic

    ii. establish the current state-of-the-art regarding research about a given topic

   iii. the highest level of evidence

B.   individual experimental studies

     i. include findings from an individual randomized controlled experimental research study, also referred to as a randomized controlled trial (RCT)

    ii. provide very high level of control for examining the probability and causality of research variables

   iii. provide even stronger recommendations when there are consistent findings from multiple individual studies

  C.   quasi-experimental studies

       i.   have less control over the research variables

      ii.   this type of study is done when experimental design cannot be used, for example, when research subjects cannot be assigned randomly to treatment conditions, such as when withholding treatment would be unethical

     iii.   this level of study leads to moderate recommendations for action

  D.   nonexperimental studies

       i.   do not have the level of control of either the experimental or quasi-experimental study

      ii.   data are collected without using controls

     iii.   merely describes the negative or positive relationships among selected variables

     iv.   this level of study usually leads to moderate recommendations for action

  E.   program evaluation

       i.   includes literature reviews

      ii.   limited evidence comes from within an institution such as benchmarking or comparing the institution's data with those from another institution

  F.   opinions of respected authorities

       i.   includes opinions from institutional research committee, a continuous quality improvement committee, or an individual expert

      ii.   there is little evidence other than the consensus of experts (cited in Rinda, 2003).

3. Current multidisciplinary **practice models**

  A.   University of Colorado hospital model

       i.   presents a framework of thinking about using different sources of information to support or change practice

      ii.   links nine sources of evidence to a research core:

         a.   benchmarking data: compare item, for example, length of stay for one patient compared with other patients with same diagnosis in the organization and other organizations nationally

         b.   cost-effective analysis: analyze cost-effectiveness of treatment(s) for a selected diagnosis, for example, hip arthroplasty

         c.   pathophysiology: review test results and laboratory findings and implications in the context of alterations in physiology that result from disease

   d. retrospective or concurrent chart review: assess changes in condition (use risk assessment scales, if needed)
   e. quality improvement and risk data: review and analyze data about patient progress and risk assessment
   f. standards (international, national, or local): assess effectiveness of care based on relevant guidelines
   g. infection control data: review any results from cultures; institute appropriate precautions and/or treatment
   h. patient preferences: discuss with the patient his or her wishes regarding directives, treatment, etc.; document and implement
   i. clinical expertise: consult nurses who have experience or training in relevant areas (for example, wound care, pain management, etc.) (University of Colorado Hospital Research Council, cited in Jadlos, 2003)

B. Concept of benchmarking

   i. **benchmarking** is the "continuous process of measuring products, services, and practices against the toughest competitors or those recognized as industry leaders" (Camp, 1994, cited in Jadlos, 2003)
   ii. for nurses, benchmarking usually occurs by comparing results to national guidelines or assessment indicators, for example:
      a. Braden Scale for Predicting Pressure Sore Risk (Bergstrom, Braden, Laguzza, & Holman, 1987)
      b. Agency for Healthcare Research and Quality (AHRQ) guidelines for prevention of pressure ulcers (1992b), treatment of pressure ulcers (AHCPR, 1994a) and national standards for managing cancer pain (1994b)
      c. Joint Commission on Accreditation of Healthcare Organizations' standard for pain assessment (1999) (also see below)

C. Model for Improvement; another model for using evidence-based practice

   i. model begins with three questions:
      a. what are we trying to accomplish?
      b. how will we know that a change is an improvement?
      c. what change can we make that will result in an improvement?
   ii. questions provide foundation for plan, do, study, act (**PDSA**) **cycle.**
      a. plan: once the questions have been identified on what needs to be improved, a multidisciplinary staff can plan how to make the improvement happen
      b. do: once the plan is in place, all staff caring for the patient, implement the plan and collect agreed-upon data (such as

patient response to interventions by collecting objective data such as level of pain, vital signs, laboratory tests, complications, and length of stay)

c. study: after collecting data for a specified time, the staff reviews the data collected

d. act: based on the data collected, the staff decides to continue the plan or alter it (Langley et al., 1996)

4. Specific practice areas currently impacted by **evidence-based practice models**

A. Pain management

i. JCAHO standard for pain assessment

ii. application of evidence-based practice model

a. based on finding that pain is a major health problem and that untreated or undertreated pain delays patient progress toward positive outcomes of care

b. standard integrates pain assessment and management into the standards that JCAHO uses to accredit health care facilities

iii. PDSA phases of model cycle

a. plan: all patients are screened at admission for presence of pain; if patients have pain, the staff obtains additional information about pain quality, intensity, frequency, and previous treatment and whether previous treatment strategies reduced pain

b. do: staff provides ongoing pain assessment, including use of more than one pain assessment tool or measure, if needed

c. study: staff ensures that all those who care for the patient are educated about pain and barriers to communicating about pain; pain assessment tools are displayed where assessments are conducted

d. act: pain management strategies are included in the care plan and modified as needed, based on the data gathered (Rinda, 2003)

B. This model is often applied to other critical areas of patient care that are responsible for increased length of stay and disproportionate use of resources; for example, pressure ulcer management and chronic wound management

i. pressure ulcer management

a. economic impact of treating pressure ulcers is significant (from $5000 to $40,000 per incident) (Phillips, 1997)

b. prevention is the most cost-effective approach

      c. the key to prevention is identification of at-risk people, using evidence-based guidelines such as *Pressure Ulcers in Adults: Prediction and Prevention*

    ii. chronic wound management

      a. the goal of wound management is to restore skin integrity and normal function

      b. injured tissue must be repaired

      c. infection control is paramount

      d. host factors such as vascular insufficiency and diabetes will delay wound healing

      e. evidence-based practice is important to achieve the best outcomes with the most cost-effective approach

5. Step-by-step process for developing new programs

    A. There are a variety of models for moving research into practice. The eight steps listed below are based on Gennaro et al. (2000):

      i. gather and organize best-level evidence

      ii. collect facts to support plans as well as alternative ideas

      iii. format evidence for change in the most convincing way possible

      iv. adapt the specific practice change for the setting (medical-surgical, critical care, perioperative)

      v. demonstrate that the change is likely to help achieve the desired results

      vi. involve stakeholders

      vii. pilot test the change

      viii. publish experiences (cited in Cooke et al., 2004)

    B. Cooke et al. note that it is also important to

      i. conduct a "needs assessment" to ensure that change is warranted and identify support needed to accomplish the change

      ii. identify barriers to implementing evidence-based practice in the organization (especially at the unit level)

    C. A Hospice and Palliative Nursing position paper (2004) cites a six-step model:

      i. assess the need for a change in practice

      ii. link problem with interventions and outcomes

      iii. synthesize best evidence

      iv. design a change in practice

      v. implement and evaluate the practice change

      vi. integrate and maintain the practice change (Rosswurm & Larrabee, 1999, cited in HPNA, 2004)

REVIEW ACTIVITIES

Questions

1. Which of the following is true about evidence-based care?
    a. it supports doing above knowing
    b. it uses the best evidence if the evidence fits current protocols
    c. it uses outcomes research to develop care strategies and delivery
    d. it requires nurses to conduct their own research

2. Which of the following is true about evidence-based nursing practice?
    a. it uses information derived from theory and research to shape nursing care
    b. it requires an organization to have a department of nursing research
    c. it does not include health professionals from other disciplines
    d. it embraces the medical model of disease

3. This type of study is done when experimental design cannot be used, for example, when research subjects cannot be assigned randomly to treatment conditions.
    a. quasi-experimental
    b. nonexperimental
    c. program evaluation
    d. individual experimental

4. This type of study provides little evidence other than the consensus of experts and is the least reliable type of study.
    a. program evaluation
    b. quasi-experimental
    c. opinion of respected authorities
    d. individual experimental

5. This type of study, which determines what the research knows about that topic, is the highest level of evidence.
    a. program evaluation
    b. meta-analysis of multiple controlled studies
    c. individual experimental
    d. quasi-experimental

6. This practice model begins with three questions (What are we trying to accomplish? How will we know that a change is an improvement? What change can we make that will result in an improvement?):
    a. Model for Improvement
    b. Braden Scale

 c. AHRQ Clinical Practice Guidelines
 d. University of Colorado model

Critical Thinking Questions

1. Traditionally, normal saline boluses have been instilled into artificial airways as part of pulmonary hygiene to thin secretions and optimize their removal. Is this practice supported by research?

2. Intravenous catheters that are used intermittently, rather than for continuous infusions, need to be flushed to maintain patency. What practice is supported by nursing research? (Include frequency of flushes and solution(s) to be used.)

3. Hydrogen peroxide has traditionally been used in health care facilities and at home alike to clean wounds. Is this practice evidence-based? Is it an appropriate practice?

4. Some over-the-counter pain relievers for headache contain caffeine in addition to the analgesic. Is this practice evidence-based or simply a marketing ploy?

Discussion Questions

1. For the health care organization with which you are most familiar, what evidence-based policies and procedures are used to guide care?

2. Can you think of areas in an organization where you have worked or done a clinical rotation that would be improved by implementing evidence-based care?

3. What would be your first step in implementing evidence-based care in your organization? Who are the key staff stakeholders? What would be the best way to communicate your ideas and objectives?

Works Cited

Agency for Health Care Policy and Research. (1992a). *Acute Pain Management: Operative or Medical Procedures and Trauma.* (Clinical Practice Guideline, Pub. No. 92-0032). Rockville, MD: Author.

Agency for Health Care Policy and Research. (1992b). *Pressure Ulcers in Aadults: Prediction and Prevention* (Clinical Practice Guideline No. 92-0047). Rockville, MD: Author.

Agency for Health Care Policy and Research. (1994a). *Management of Cancer Pain* (Clinical Practice Guideline No. 94-0592). Rockville, MD: Author.

Agency for Health Care Policy and Research. (1994b). *Treatment of Ppressure Ulcers* (Clinical Practice Guideline No. 94-0652). Rockville, MD: Author.

Bellack, J. P., & O'Neil, E. H. (2000). Recreating nursing practice for a new century: Recommendations and implications of the Pew Health Professions Commission's final report. *Nursing Health Care Perspectives, 21*(1), 14–21.

Bergstrom, N., Braden, B. J., Laguzza, A., & Holman, V. (1987). The Braden Scale for Predicting Pressure Sore Risk. *Nursing Research, 36*(4), 205–210.

Bryant, L. (1998). The ontology of the discipline of nursing. *Nursing Science Quarterly, 11*, 145–146.

Camp, R., (1994). Benchmarking applied to healthcare. *The Joint Commission on Quality Improvement, 20*, 229–238.

Cooke, L., Smith-Idell, C., Dean, G., Gemmill, R., Steingass, S., Sun, V., et al. (2004). "Research to practice": A practical program to enhance the use of evidence-based practice at the unit level. *Oncology Nursing Forum, 31*(4), 825–831.

Clancy, C., & Eisenberg, J. (1998). Outcomes research: Measure the end results of health care. *Science, 282*, 245–246.

Gennaro, S., Hodnett, E., & Kearney, M. (2001). Making evidence-based practice a reality in your institution. *American Journal of Maternal Child Nursing, 26*, 236–244.

Hospice and Palliative Nurses Association. HPNA position paper available at http://www.hpna.org/pdf/Position_EvidenceBasedPractice.pdf. *Journal of Hospital and Palliative Nursing, 6*(3), 189–190.

Ingersoll, G. L. (2000). Evidence-based nursing: What it is and what it isn't. *Nursing Outlook, 48*, 151–152.

Jadlos, M. A. (2003). Strategies to improve patient care outcomes. In P. Kelly-Heidenthal (Ed.), *Nursing leadership & management* (pp. 398–427). Clifton Park, NY: Thomson Delmar Learning.

Joint Commission on Accreditation of Healthcare Organizations. (1999). *Comprehensive Accreditation Manual for Hospitals: The Official Handbook*, PE-8.

Langley, K. M., Nolan, T. W., Norman, C. L., & Provost, L. P. (1996). *A practical approach to enhancing organizational performance.* San Francisco: Jossey-Bass.

Phillips, T. J. (1997). *Cost effectiveness in wound care: A clinical source book for healthcare professionals* (pp. 367–372). Wayne, PA: Health Management Publications.

Rinda, A. (2003). Evidence-based health care. In P. Kelly-Heidenthal (Ed.), *Nursing leadership & management* (pp. 59–73). Clifton Park, NY: Thomson Delmar Learning.

Rosswurm, M. A., & Larrabee, J. H. (1999). Model for change to evidence-based practice. *Image: The Journal of Nursing Scholarship, 31*(4), 317–322.

Sackett, D. L., Rosenberg, W. M., Gray, J. A., Haynes, R. B., & Richardson, W. S. (1996). Evidence based medicine: What it is and what it isn't. *British Medical Journal, 312*(7023), 71–72.

Stetler, C. B., Morsi, D., Rucki, S., Broughton, S., Corrigan, B., Fitzgerald, J., et al. (1998). Utilization-focused integrative reviews in a nursing service. *Applied Nursing Research, 11*(4), 195–206.

Additional Resources

Geanellos, R. (2004). Nursing based evidence: Moving beyond evidence-based practice in mental health nursing. *Journal of Evaluation in Clinical Practice, 10*(2), 177–187.

Gosling, A. S., Westbrook, J. I., & Spencer, R. (2004). Nurses' use of online clinical evidence. *Journal of Advanced Nursing, 47*(2), 201–212.

Rycroft-Malone, J., Seers, K., Titchen, A., Harvey, G., Kitson, A., & McCormack, B. (2004). What counts as evidence in evidence-based practice? *Journal of Advanced Nursing, 47*(1), 81–91.

Singh, N. N., & Oswald, D. P. (2004). Evidence-based practice. Part I: General methodology. *Journal of Child & Family Studies, 13*(2), 129–143.

Singh, N. N., & Oswald, D. P. (2004). Evidence-Based Practice. Part II: A Specific Methodology. *Journal of Child & Family Studies, 13*(3), 255–263.

Veeramah, V. (2004). Utilization of research findings by graduate nurses and midwives. *Journal of Advanced Nursing, 47*(2), 183–192.

Web Sites

American Academy of Pain Management
   http://www.aapainmanage.org

Applied Nursing Research
   http://www.us.elsevierhealth.com/product.jsp?isbn=08971897

Evidence-Based Nursing, Resources McGill University Health Centre
   http://www.muhc-ebn.mcgill.ca/

Evidence-Based Nursing, University of Minnesota
   http://evidence.ahc.umn.edu/ebn.htm

Graduate Research in Nursing
   http://www.graduateresearch.com/RNPTOCPage.htm

JCAHO
   http://www.jcaho.org

Journal of Evidence Based Nursing (EBN online)
   http://ebn.bmjjournals.com

Online Journal of Knowledge Synthesis for Nursing
   http://www.stti.iupui.edu/VirginiaHendersonLibrary/OJKSNMenu.aspx

Virginia Henderson International Nursing Library (includes Registry of Nursing Research)
   http://www.stti.iupui.edu/VirginiaHendersonLibrary

Worldviews on Evidence-based Nursing
   http://www.blackwellpublishing.com/journal.asp?ref=1545-102X

14

MANAGING PATIENT CARE AND OUTCOMES THROUGH IMPROVING ORGANIZATION QUALITY

KEY TERMS

customers
FOCUS methodology
magnet status
organizational structure
outcomes monitoring
ownership
PDCA cycle
performance improvement

processes
quality assurance
quality improvement
regulatory requirements
sentinel event
system
total quality management (TQM)

INTRODUCTION

Health care organizations need to continually monitor their services to improve quality of care. The concepts of quality assurance and quality improvement (QI) began in the manufacturing industry, but QI is applicable to health care as well. This chapter discusses the key role of quality improvement in health care organizations and the different methods used to measure and improve health care processes.

KEY POINTS

1. What is **quality improvement**?

   A. Definition

      i. a systematic process to improve outcomes based on customers' needs

    ii. a proactive approach that emphasizes "doing the right thing" for the customer

    iii. became a part of health care in the 1980s when competition as well as pressure from managed care organizations and other payers to reduce cost and improve quality of care increased

    iv. is more of an overall management approach rather than a single "program"

B. History. Quality improvement has evolved from the following:

    i. **quality assurance**

      a. emerged in the 1950s, about the same time as hospital accrediting organizations

      b. began as hospital inspections, to ensure that they maintained minimum standards of care

      c. QA departments evolved into organizational mechanisms for measuring performance as well as for reporting incidents and errors

      d. QA methods: chart audits for selected patient diagnoses or procedures

      e. drawbacks were that this "after the fact" analysis did little to proactively identify problems or sustain meaningful change and in many cases, data were collected and reported in a punitive fashion without regard to whether a particular "deficiency" had an impact on patient outcomes

    ii. **performance improvement**, which focused on the manufacturing industry in the 1950s

    iii. **total quality management** (TQM)

      a. adopted by the Japanese after World War II to transform their industrial development

      b. characterized by customer/client focus, total organizational involvement, use of quality tools and statistics for measurement, and identification of key processes for improvement (Sullivan & Decker, 2001)

C. Difference between quality assurance and quality improvement

    i. focus on quality assurance (also called "doing it right")

      a. assess or measure performance

      b. determine whether performance meets standards (goal in manufacturing, for example, is "zero defects")

      c. improve performance when it does not meet standards

    ii. focus on quality improvement (also called "doing the right thing")

      a. meet the customer's needs

      b. build quality performance into the work process

      c. assess the work process to identify opportunities for improved performance

   d. employ a scientific approach to assessment and problem solving
   e. improve performance continuously as an ongoing manage-
      ment strategy, not just when standards are not met (McLaughlin
      & Houston, 2003)
   f. performance integrates processes and outcomes and continu-
      ally seeks a better way to accomplish desired outcomes

D. Principles in action in an organization

   i. **organizational structure**
      a. to maximize QI efforts
      b. needs to be flexible and able to implement changes, especially
         in rapidly changing health care environment
      c. structure needs to emphasize accountability for all people
         involved
      d. must be able to communicate effectively through different lev-
         els of staff and administrators
   ii. **outcomes monitoring**
      a. the measurement of patient response to the organizational
         structure and process
      b. measure actual clinical progress
      c. can be short term (for example, average length of patient stay)
         or long term (for example, patient survival or complication
         rate for 1, 3, or 5 years after treatment)
      d. monitoring outcomes allows an organization to study the out-
         comes and identify possible areas of concern (for example,
         postsurgical infection rates) (McLaughlin & Houston, 2003)

2. General principles of quality improvement

   A. Priority is to benefit patients and other internal and external **customers**

      i. customer is anyone who receives the output of efforts
      ii. internal customer works within the organization (for example,
          nurses in the intensive care unit are customers of radiologic tech-
          nologists using portable equipment in the unit for radiographs)
      iii. external customer is anyone outside the organization who receives
           the output of the organization (for example, patients, insurance
           companies, regulators, and the community; surgeons who bring
           patients to a hospital for surgery are also customers of the hospital)

   B. Organizations achieve quality through the participation of everyone in
      that organization; this promotes **ownership** so that employees

      i. take responsibility for an organization's success or failure
      ii. take an active role in developing new ways of doing business and
          bringing in new customers

     iii. know that their efforts are valued

     iv. for example, a nurse organizes her day so that she can spend a few moments with a critically ill patient's family; or a respiratory therapist checks with the nurse so as to coordinate treatment times for patients with chronic obstructive pulmonary disease to reduce patient fatigue

C.   Focusing on work process provides opportunities for improvement

     i. **processes** are causes or conditions that repeatedly come together in a series of steps to transfer inputs into outcomes (Langley et al., 1996)

     ii. steps in a process can be studied, based on evidence-based practice, eliminated, changed, or standardized to improve the overall work process

     iii. for example, all the steps required to take a patient's blood sample can be observed, analyzed, compared with best practices, and changed to eliminate repetition of steps or otherwise improve speed and accuracy of results

D.   Decisions to change or improve a **system** are based on data

     i. a system is an interdependent group of items, people, or processes with a common purpose (Langley, et al., 1996)

     ii. outcomes can be observed and improved on, by analyzing their systemic roots

     iii. for example, to improve the time required to take a patient's blood sample and receive diagnostic results, you would need not only to improve the response time of the phlebotomist, but also examine the processes at work in the lab

E.   Improvement of service quality is a continuous process (McLaughlin & Houston, 2003)

     i. products or services are designed and made based on the knowledge about the customer

     ii. the customer judges the product or service and how well it does or does not meet his/her needs

     iii. based on this information, the product or service is improved (Sullivan & Decker, 2001; McLaughlin & Houston, 2003)

3. Quality improvement for patient care measured by overall value of care

A.   Value as function of outcomes and cost

     i. value is the quality of an outcome or outcomes divided by the cost required to achieve those outcomes

      ii. outcomes can be measured according to clinical standards or patient satisfaction standards

     iii. costs include

        a. direct costs: the cost of actual patient care, such as medications, equipment, and direct patient caregiver salaries

        b. indirect costs: the cost of activities or services such as electricity, or salaries of administrative staff not directly involved in patient care

B.   Quality improvement occurs due to

      i. standardizing care delivery processes, which decrease the cost of care

     ii. using evidence-based principles, which improve care outcomes (McLaughlin & Houston, 2003) (See Chapter 13)

4. Strategies for quality improvement

A.   **PDCA** (plan, do, check, act) **cycle**

      i. begins with three questions:

        a. what are we trying to accomplish?

        b. how will we know that a change is an improvement?

        c. what changes can we make that will result in improvement?

     ii. *plan:* develop a change, test, or activity aimed at improvement

    iii. *do:* carry the change or test out, preferably on a small scale

    iv. *check:* study the results to evaluate what was learned and what can be predicted

     v. *act:* adopt the change, send it through the cycle again, under different conditions, or abandon the idea

B.   **FOCUS methodology** includes five steps for moving through an improvement process

      i. *focus* on an improvement idea

        a. key to this step is to ask, "What is the problem?"

        b. articulate the opportunity for improvement and obtain data to support the hypothesis that an opportunity exists

     ii. *organize* a team that knows the process

        a. identify staff who directly participate in the process since they will understand it best

        b. identify a team leader

    iii. *clarify* what is happening in the current process

        a. use a flow diagram to illustrate processes

        b. analyze macro level of process to identify too many steps in a process, areas that are not well defined or understood, long wait times between processes, or multiple paths that indicate too many people involved (too many people delivering services to a patient, for example, waste time and confuse the patient)

    c. analyze micro levels of process, including examining decision points, redundancy of processes, waiting time areas, rework loops, and handoffs

  iv. *understand* the degree of change needed

    a. team can review data gathered, literature on the topic, and competitive benchmarks

    b. how are other organizations doing this process?

  v. *solve* the problem

    a. select a solution for improvement that involves the staff directly involved

    b. use an implementation plan to check progress of solution

    c. identify activity to be completed, who is responsible for it, and when it will be done

C. Benchmarking

  i. measuring and comparing the results of key work processes with those of "best performers" in a field or industry

  ii. is a collaborative and ongoing measurement process

  iii. will identify gaps in performance and provide options for improvement

  iv. focuses on key services or processes; for example, length of time in the OR for a surgical procedure, or length of postoperative in-patient stay

D. **Regulatory requirements**

  i. Joint Commission on Accreditation of Healthcare Organizations (JCAHO) has developed standards to guide critical activities that health care organizations perform

  ii. preparing for an accreditation survey gives a health care organization a wealth of data and information, which can be used to begin improvement strategies

E. Review when sentinel event occurs

  i. an adverse **sentinel event** is an unexpected occurrence causing death or serious physical or psychological injury to a patient (JCAHO, 1998)

  ii. analysis of these events provides opportunities for improving the system

  iii. linking sentinel event review to the organization's performance improvement system will identify strategies to prevent future sentinel events

      iv. an example of a sentinel event is wrong site surgery—typically operating on the wrong side of the body

         a. health care organizations studying these sentinel events realized that no standards for preoperative marking or validation existed

         b. analyzing these events and identifying strategies to prevent future events led to standardization of this protocol and JCAHO requirements now call for using a skin marker to identify the correct site for surgery

      v. key to sentinel event program is to share information among all accredited health care organizations so as to reduce the risk in which the event will recur

F. Balanced scorecard concept

      i. the main concept is that progress measurement has to be balanced between medical, patient satisfaction, and cost outcomes

      ii. any change in one area must be evaluated as to how it affects the balance in another area

      iii. this measurement method evaluates the following four key areas

         a. functional status of patient

         b. clinical status of patient

         c. patient satisfaction

         d. cost of care (McLaughlin & Houston, 2003)

5. Gathering and sharing information about quality improvement

A. Using storyboard to share information

      i. visually outlines the progress in major steps of improvement methodology

      ii. can be displayed in high traffic areas of a department to inform all staff of QI efforts under way

      iii. can communicate a completed process or illustrate a process that is under way

B. Using patient satisfaction data in determining quality improvement

      i. via questionnaire

         a. asks patients how they felt about health care encounter (patient satisfaction survey)

         b. can be compared or benchmarked with other data

         c. requires that different departments or organizations use the same data collection tools

      ii. via focus group or postcare interview conducted after the patients' discharge

      iii. most reliable data come from third party organizations that provide the service so that data are not generated within the organization and subject to adjustments

         a. many third-party organizations will benchmark to other health care providers of the same size or other demographics used for comparison

C. Types of data used to examine quality improvement efforts

    i. time series data

      a. allows QI team to see changes in quality over time

      b. allows team to differentiate between actual changes and normal fluctuations

    ii. other charts that can be used: fishbone diagrams (also called cause and effect diagrams), which allow staff to see that most problems have multiple causes or roots, Pareto charts, or control charts (also called a check sheet) (McLaughlin & Houston, 2003)

D. Magnet hospitals

    i. **magnet status** is the highest level of recognition that an organization can achieve for its nursing department

      a. awarded after the organization has completed a rigorous application process and passed an on-site visit by examiners

      b. the organization must renew its magnet status regularly

    ii. benefits of becoming a magnet hospital

      a. recognition of staff expertise and ability

      b. increased employee recruitment and retention

      c. competitive advantages versus other nonmagnet institutions

      d. creates a "magnet culture" and creates high staff morale

      e. improves patient quality outcomes (JCAHO news release, American Nurses Credentialing Center)

    iii. not everyone is sold on the magnet concept; many nursing unions have expressed concerns that achieving magnet designation is another costly review process that focuses on process, and not necessarily on outcomes or working conditions. This is an area that will no doubt continue to be debated well into the future.

REVIEW ACTIVITIES

Questions

1. A systematic process to improve outcomes based on customers' needs is called

a. quality assurance
b. quality improvement
c. total quality management
d. organizational structure

2. Which of the following is not a characteristic of quality improvement?
   a. meeting the customer's needs
   b. building quality performance into work process
   c. assessing work process to identify opportunities for downsizing
   d. improving performance continuously as an ongoing management strategy

3. The measurement of clinical progress and patient response to organizational structure and process is called
   a. organizational structure
   b. ownership
   c. outcomes monitoring
   d. total quality management

4. A goal of "zero defects" is one characteristic of
   a. quality assurance
   b. quality improvement
   c. benchmarking
   d. outcomes monitoring

5. Cause or condition that repeatedly comes together in a series of steps to transfer inputs into outcomes is called a(n)
   a. system
   b. outcome
   c. process
   d. customer

6. A system is
   a. a process to improve outcomes based on customer needs
   b. measure of patient response to clinical progress
   c. causes or conditions that come together to transfer inputs into outcomes
   d. an interdependent group of items, people, or processes with a common purpose.

7. In the PDCA cycle for quality improvement, the letters stand for plan, do, check, and
   a. account
   b. act
   c. alleviate
   d. ask

8. Which of the following is true about benchmarking?
   a. it measures and compares key work processes with those of the best performers in an industry
   b. it requires a one-time expenditure of time and money
   c. it does not apply to indicators affected by patient variables
   d. it is generally not useful for core products and services

9. Sentinel events are
   a. expected
   b. useful for improving an organization's system
   c. always reported to JCAHO
   d. an indicator of magnet status

Critical Thinking Questions

1. Wrong site surgery is one of the JCAHO patient care safety initiatives. There are seven National Patient Safety Goals for hospitals. What are they? For one of the goals, describe the steps an organization could take to improve its quality indicators in this area.

2. Using the PDCA model, identify ways by which a patient's blood sample could be mislabeled with a different patient's name. Then describe a process that would assure that a patient's blood sample is not mislabeled.

Discussion Questions

1. What quality improvement initiatives have been taken in the organization in which you work or in which you have recently done a clinical rotation? What areas did the QI focus on? What were the results?

2. Choose a hospital in which you work or have recently done a clinical rotation. What would that organization need to do to be ready to apply for magnet status? Do you work at or know of an organization that has gone through this process? Interview a nursing leader in that organization to learn what benefits the organization has derived from achieving magnet status.

3. Choose an organization in which you work or have done a clinical rotation. What processes or services would be useful to benchmark?

4. Choose a unit on which you work or have done a clinical rotation. For that unit, what indicators are monitored most closely? What is the rationale for choosing those indicators?

Works Cited

Benefits of becoming a magnet designated facility. American Nurses Credentialing Center. Accessed August 9, 2004 at: http://www.nursingworld.org/ancc/magnet/benes.html.

Dartmouth-Hitchcock wins "Magnet" status recognized for top quality nursing environment. (2004). *Nursing News* (New Hampshire), *28*(1), 1, 3.

Joint Commission on Accreditation of Healthcare Organizations. (1998). *Comprehensive accreditation manual for hospitals.* Oakbrook, IL: Author.

McLaughlin, M., & Houston, K. (2003). Managing outcomes using an organizational quality improvement model. In P. Kelly-Heidenthal (Ed.), *Nursing leadership & management* (pp. 376–397). Clifton Park, NY: Thomson Delmar Learning.

Sullivan, E. J., & Decker, P. J. (2001). *Effective leadership and management in nursing* (5th ed.). Upper Saddle River, NJ: Prentice Hall.

Taylor, N. T. (2004). The magnetic pull. *Nurse Manager*, *35*(4), 59–60, 62–69.

Additional Resources

Crosby, P. B. (1989). *Let's talk quality.* New York: McGraw-Hill.

Deming, W. E. (1986). *Out of the crisis.* Cambridge, MA: Center for Advanced Engineering Study.

Joint Commission on Accreditation of Healthcare Organizations. *Facts about patient safety.* Available online at: http://www.jcaho.org/accredited+organizations/patient+safety/facts+about+patient+safety.htm Last accessed September 14, 2004.

New Magnet Facilities. (2004). *American Journal of Nursing*, *104*(3), 22.

Trofino, A. J. (2000). Transformational leadership: Moving total quality management to world-class organizations. *International Nursing Review*, *47*(4), 232–243.

Gessell, S. B., & Gregory, N. (2004). Identifying priority actions for improving patient satisfaction with outpatient cancer care. *Journal of Nursing Care Quality*, *19*(3), 226–234.

Scott-Cawiezel, J., Schenkman, M., Moore, L., Vojir, C., Connolly, R. P., Pratt, M., et al. Exploring nursing home staff's perceptions of communication and leadership to facilitate quality improvement. *Journal of Nursing Care Quality*, *19*(3), 242–253.

Morrison, M. H., Cheng, R. A., & Lee, R. H. (2004). Best-practices protocols can improve quality. *Nursing Homes Long Term Care Management*, *53*(6), 64–68.

Web Sites

Agency for Healthcare Research and Quality: *Quality Information and Improvement* http://www.ahcpr.gov/qual/qualix.htm

American Nurses Credentialing Center: Magnet Hospital
http://www.nursingworld.org/ancc/magnet/benes.html

Baldrige National Quality Program
http://www.quality.nist.gov/index.html

Institute for Healthcare Improvement (IHI) (benchmarking data)
http://www.ihi.org/ihi

Morbidity & Mortality Rounds on the Web
http://www.webmm.ahrq.gov/

National Guidelines Clearinghouse
http://www.guidelines.gov

Press Ganey Associates, Inc.: Patient Satisfaction
http://www.pressganey.com/client_recognition

15 MANAGING AND SUPPORTING EXCELLENCE IN STAFF PERFORMANCE

adult learners

care delivery models

case management

clinical pathways

clinical skills

full-time equivalent (FTE)

interpersonal skills

job performance

mentor

motivation

networking

nursing hours per patient day

partnership

performance measurement

staff performance

staffing

technical skills

INTRODUCTION

Nurse leaders who are managers not only need to make sure that enough employees are available to meet patient care objectives, but also to see that employees' performance is observed, assessed, evaluated, and corrected when necessary. This chapter discusses key concepts about employee or staff performance, and suggests ways that nurse managers can help employees function to the best of their abilities.

KEY POINTS

1. Definition

    A. **Staff performance** usually includes the following:

        i. daily job performance according to requirements of job description

       ii. attendance

     iii. punctuality

      iv. adherence to organization policies and procedures
      v. absence of errors, incidents, or accidents
      vi. honesty and trustworthiness (both to staff and patients/clients) (Sullivan & Decker, 2001)

B. Leadership's role in staff's **job performance**
      i. helping team members reach their full potential
      ii. recognizing that the success of the organization depends on the people who work for the organization
      iii. nurse leader/manager shall
          a. figure out what it takes to do the job
          b. define job requirements
          c. determine the personnel, and their skills and attitudes, which can accomplish the job (Costello-Nickitas, 1997)

C. Staff performance is developed on three levels

      i. **clinical skills**
          a. specialized knowledge and judgment used to diagnose and treat human responses to health problems and to support licensed and noncredentialed staff in this area
      ii. **technical skills**
          a. analytical ability and competence in using equipment and carrying out procedures specific to nursing care
          b. managers must be able to assess staff skills, as well as improve them
          c. managers must also be able to redirect and motivate team members so that they remain competent and confident in the care they give
      iii. **interpersonal skills**
          a. connecting the tasks that must be accomplished with the human side of people performing the tasks while focusing on patient needs
          b. enabling communication, consideration, and cooperation (Costello-Nickitas, 1997)

D. Leadership as partnership

      i. **partnership:** "a desired relationship between two parties seeking to work together toward a common goal" (Costello-Nickitas, 1997, p. 108)
      ii. both parties must be willing to assess themselves and their attributes
      iii. self-assessment and introspection allow team members to empathize with other staff and with patients/clients

E. Effective nurse leaders/managers develop a personnel focus that is attuned to staff, patient, and market needs

      i. monitoring and facilitating personnel productivity and development
- a. ask team members what they want and need
- b. provide appropriate, up-to-date training focusing on need-to-know information
- c. encourage mentoring
- d. be a role model

      ii. understanding patient requirements and needs
- a. develop a strategic quality plan to promote nursing quality (see chapter 14)
- b. design or improve training requirements to meet these demands
- c. promote teamwork
- d. benchmark nursing services (Costello-Nickitas, 1997)

      iii. strategic focus on quality
- a. ask customers and staff for feedback and information
- b. empower staff to solve problems; give them authority to do so
- c. remember that even small improvements can produce large results (not every change has to be a "major" project)
- d. involve everyone in the quality focus, not just certain staff levels (Gouillart & Sturdivant, 1994)

      iv. understanding and meeting the organization's vision, mission, and objectives
- a. ensure that all personnel understand the organization's objectives
- b. based on organization's objectives, put the right personnel in the right place to meet these objectives
- c. instill a can-do attitude in the personnel
- d. encourage creativity and "outside the box" thinking to meet objectives (Costello-Nickitas, 1997)

F. What motivates employees? According to Sullivan and Decker (2001, p. 301), the key **motivation** factors are:

      i. employee needs, goals, and abilities
      ii. job design
      iii. leadership style
      iv. benefits
      v. compensation
      vi. recruitment and selection processes

2. Strategies for developing staff excellence

A. Mentoring

      i. second only to education in importance for staff development

      ii. a **mentor** is a "more experienced role model who guides, coaches, and advises the less experienced" (Vance & Olson, 1991, cited in Costello-Nickitas, 1997, p. 112)

     iii. mentor gives professional advice, helps avoid pitfalls, and arranges introductions to the larger network

     iv. mentors also provide
- a. opportunities for career development and advancement
- b. encouragement and professional support
- c. recognition of potential and effort
- d. opportunities for professional and personal growth
- e. a working example of leadership and other role modeling

B. Networking

      i. **networking** is a method of connecting with other people and resources that provides
- a. access to crucial information and contacts
- b. avenues for identifying useful people and maintaining contacts with them
- c. expanding one's opportunities by being able to work with contacts of others in the network

     ii. networking may be informal or formal
- a. exchanging handshakes or business cards (informal)
- b. joining professional nursing organizations, business organizations (such as chambers of commerce), etc

     iii. to be successful networkers, nurse leaders need to
- a. network regularly
- b. get to know people both inside and outside the organization
- c. be good communicators (both effective listening and speaking skills)
- d. be prepared (keep cards on hand, take notes on contact information, etc.) (Costello-Nickitas, 1997)
- e. always keep in mind that for networking to be successful, one must provide contacts and assistance as well as get contacts and assistance

C. Understand needs of **adult learners**. Adults learn differently from people of school age. An effective nurse manager can build staff performance by ensuring that the training and professional continuing education programs are designed to meet the needs of adult learners.

      i. Four stages of adult learning
- a. have an experience; for example, perform a patient procedure, such as maintaining a chest tube
- b. reflect on the experience; for example, go over the steps required to assess the patient and the drainage tube; then review the steps taken to maintain the drainage system

     c. relate the experience to a mental model or theory; for example, theories about suction rate, positive and negative pressures

     d. plan what to do next; for example, monitor the drain more frequently or stop suction so that the patient can get out of bed and walk

  ii. Focus on the learner's preferred style, which corresponds to one of the four adult learning stages listed above

     a. active: prefer to learn by doing (allow these learners time and space to actually touch the equipment and go through the procedure steps initially in simulation)

     b. reflective: prefer to learn by thinking about or observing experiences (allow these learners to watch someone else perform the procedure first, then allow time for them to think about what they saw and relate it to their previous experiences)

     c. theorist: prefer to learn by thoroughly understanding the theory or model that underlies a concept (allow these learners to study or review information on the physics of drainage and suction)

     d. pragmatists: prefer to learn by planning or envisioning the "what's next" (allow these learners to "troubleshoot" the next procedure by planning and outlining action steps) (Reynolds, 2002)

     e. it is important to remember that most people can use more than one learning style, depending on circumstances, but most show a strong preference for one style

  iii. McCarthy's 4-MAT model. This theory suggests that, in order to learn, adults need to answer four questions:

     a. what? (for example: What is this procedure? What does it do? What equipment is needed? Is sterile technique required or not?)

     b. why? (for example: Why are we performing this procedure? How will it benefit the patient? Does it treat an existing problem or prevent a different problem or complication?)

     c. how? (for example: What steps must be completed to perform the procedure properly? What precautions need to be observed? What supplies and personnel are needed?)

     d. what if? (for example: What should we do if the procedure does not go as planned? What if the patient objects?) (cited in Reynolds, 2002)

  iv. Neuro-linguistic programming. This adult learning theory says that most people prefer one of the following learning styles:

     a. visual (learn best through seeing pictures, images, or words, for example, videos of procedure steps, outlines of procedure, texts, and illustrations)

     b. auditory (learn best through sounds and the spoken word, for example, lecture from an instructor, conversations with other caregivers, Q&A sessions, listening to books on tape)

    c. kinesthetic (learn best through performing tasks and physical interaction; for example, supervised tasks, using models) (Reynolds, 2002)

  v. Other factors

    a. intelligence is not just mathematical and verbal; Gardner (1983) emphasized a wide range of "intelligences" that include not only math and verbal skills, but also musical, bodily-kinesthetic, interpersonal, spatial, and inter- and intrapersonal abilities

    b. much of the adult learning research has taken place in the United States and the United Kingdom; however, all learning and training must take into account the multicultural nature of the current workplace (VanDerWall, 1998)

3. Staffing needs

  A. Meeting **staffing** needs of an organization. To accurately and effectively plan for care, the nurse manager needs to know the following:

    i. staff knowledge and experience

    ii. the severity of patients' illnesses

    iii. the amount of nursing time available

    iv. the care delivery model that the organization follows

    v. care management tools in place

    vi. what the health care organization provides to support and facilitate patient care

  B. Effectively determining staffing needs. To determine staffing needs, the nurse manager needs to know full time equivalents (FTE) and nursing hours per patient day (NHPPD):

    i. **full-time equivalent (FTE):** the measure of work commitment of a full-time employee

    a. an FTE who works 40 hours per week is referred to as 1.0 FTE

    b. 1.0 FTE means a person works 5 days a week, 8 hours a day (40 hours/week), for 52 weeks each year (total of 2,080 hours)

    c. FTE is further divided into productive hours (hours worked and available for patient care) and nonproductive hours (benefit time such as sick time, vacation, and education/training)

    d. FTE calculations for staffing must include only productive time (FTE hours minus nonproductive hours)

    ii. **nursing hours per patient day** (NHPPD)

    a. standard measure that quantifies the nursing time available to each patient per nursing staff member

    b. only productive hours are calculated

    c. for example, for one 24-hour period, a unit has 20 patients, with 5 nursing staff available on each shift (15 total staff x 8 hour

shifts) which equals 120 nursing hours available for 20
patients, or 6 hours per patient (Bernat, 2003)

C. How to evaluate staffing effectiveness? It is the nurse manager's ongoing responsibility to monitor staff effectiveness to define, measure, and
review outcomes.

    i. patient outcomes. An American Nurses Association study con-
firms the relationship between nursing staffing and patient outcomes. Nurse staffing most strongly affected outcomes for
      a. pneumonia (incidence and length of stay)
      b. postoperative infections
      c. pressure ulcers
      d. urinary tract infections (Lichtig, Knaug, Rison-McCoy, &
         Wozniak, 2000)
    Outcomes are negatively affected when nurse staffing and skill
mix are inadequate.

    ii. nursing outcomes
      a. it is also important for the nurse manager to track staff percep-
tions about staffing adequacy
      b. staff need to have both verbal and written ways to report
staffing concerns
      c. inadequate NHPPD are associated with negative changes in
patient acuity and medication errors (Bernat, 2003)

4. Management tools for care delivery. Different organizations use different
models and tools to manage the delivery of care. These include:

A. **Clinical pathways**
    i. outlines the expected clinical course and timed outcomes for a
specific diagnosis or surgical procedure recovery, such as a joint
arthroplasty
    ii. take a different form in each organization that develops them
    iii. are done day by day, with daily expected outcomes for the patient
    iv. pathways may include multidisciplinary orders, such as those
from physicians and physical therapists, in addition to nursing
plans to provide a comprehensive picture of patient progress
    v. many organizations provide patients with a version of the pathway
so that they know what is expected of them during their recovery

B. **Case management**
    i. strategy to improve care and reduce costs by coordinating care
    ii. case manager is typically assigned to monitor and coordinate
various areas of care to meet established goals from time of

      admission to discharge and to make sure nothing "falls through the cracks"

  iii. case management function can be provided by the RN at the bedside, but complex cases (for example, a multiple trauma patient) may require a dedicated case manager

C. Current **care delivery models**

    i. case method: the oldest model for nursing care delivery in which one nurse provides care for one or more patient(s) (depending on acuity)

   ii. total patient care: the contemporary version of the case method—the nurse is responsible for total patient care for that shift. RNs are responsible for several patients and are assisted by other licensed personnel (such as LPNs) or noncredentialed assistive personnel.

  iii. functional nursing: divides the nursing work into functional units that are assigned to team members, such as designating one nurse to administer medications

  iv. team nursing: assigns staff to teams that are responsible for a group of patients. Each team is led by a registered nurse, who supervises and coordinates care, and provides professional direction to team members.

   v. primary nursing: clearly delineates the RN's responsibility and accountability and designates the RN as the primary care provider. Primary nursing is made up of four elements:
     a. allocation and acceptance of individual responsibility by one person
     b. assigning daily patient care via the case method system
     c. direct person-to-person communication
     d. one person operationally responsible for care quality on a unit (Manthey, 1980)

  vi. patient-focused care: focuses on patient needs rather than staffing issues. Usually all patient services are decentralized and staffing is based on the patient's care needs. However, some suggest that this term is used as a subterfuge to hide the fact that there are fewer RN staff members and more noncredentialed personnel performing patient care activities.

  vii. differentiated practice: sorts the roles, functions, and work of RNs according to criteria such as education, clinical experience, or competence (Baker et al., 1997)

  viii. patient care redesign: in response to cost-reduction mandates, care is reorganized to maintain care quality, while reducing costs of providing care; usually depends on extensive use of noncredentialed assistive personnel, without review of RN care required (Bernat, 2003)

D. Supporting staff excellence through **performance measurement**. According to Costello-Nickitas (1997), the only way to know whether the staff are meeting their goals is to measure performance.

    i. purpose of performance measurement is to
       a. provide feedback
       b. justify merit increases and other compensation adjustments
       c. identify candidates for promotion
       d. confirm hiring decisions
       e. counsel and terminate

    ii. to effectively assess employee performance, the nurse manager must know the principles of performance management
       a. know the job description and performance standards for the person being evaluated
       b. remain objective and evaluate performance over time, not just the month before the formal performance appraisal is due
       c. encourage employee to set attainable short-term and long-term goals and to include professional development activities
       d. allow the person being evaluated to respond to the evaluation and discuss any performance successes or difficulties
       e. identify specific ways for employee to improve job performance and specific ways to motivate employee
       f. write down goals and objectives in a contract that specifies expectations and encourages growth

    iii. the key elements of performance measurement
       a. quality and volume of work. Does the person perform the amount of work expected and do it according to standards set by the department?
       b. work knowledge. Does the employee understand department policies and procedures, regulations, resources, and trends that are applicable to his or her daily responsibilities?
       c. work judgment. Does the person show reliable and consistent decision making and predictable, appropriate behavior?
       d. organization. Does the person effectively plan and organize work, and meet set deadlines and use time wisely?
       e. responsibility and flexibility. Does the employee accept responsibility for his or her work and avoid blaming others for failures? Does he or she accept instruction or direction appropriately? Can the employee readily adapt to changing conditions such as admissions, changes in patient condition, and other modifications to do the assignment during a given shift?
       f. interpersonal skills. Does the employee communicate effectively with other staff members, patients, families, etc.?

5. Roles and responsibilities of the nurse manager in evaluating staff performance

A. Six key activities
   i. set specific expectations (behaviors that are expected of the employee)
   ii. encourage balance between performance measurements and standards of care to facilitate setting measurable goals and ensure that employees take personal responsibility for meeting goals
   iii. review goals and action plans with staff to facilitate feedback cycle
   iv. reassess systems and resources needed to obtain goals, and work with staff to determine priorities and alternatives
   v. follow work progress (nurse manager acts as motivator and problem-solver when challenges arise; manager reinforces prior employee achievements and helps employees find new ways to meet or exceed expectations)
   vi. encourage or reinforce achievement (Costello-Nickitas, 1997; Bernat, 2003)

B. The importance of job descriptions as part of performance measurement
   i. job descriptions help nurse managers produce results such as customer satisfaction, an efficient and effective work environment, meeting patient care objectives, and cost-effective care
   ii. effective job descriptions
      a. help employees understand their duties
      b. improve work flow
      c. evaluate job performance
      d. clarify relationships among jobs
      e. identify potential training needs
      f. help determine employee hiring and placement needs
      g. establish a structure for promotion and salaries (Costello-Nickitas, 1997)
      h. are consistent with licensure laws and do not assign duties to noncredentialed staff that can only be performed by licensed nurses

C. Additional performance tools
   i. using feedback for performance management
      a. anecdotal notes to record behaviors of employees being evaluated
      b. supportive counseling to provide feedback to employee about job performance
      c. feedback should be a regular part of employee/supervisor communication, both in the context of formal evaluations and informally throughout the workday

ii. rewarding successful performance. A variety of rewards (which must always be linked to performance) are available to nurse managers:

    a. incentives (for example, lunch provided by nurse manager)

    b. recognition (for example, "employee of the week" picture prominently displayed)

    c. promotion

    d. choice of preferences, such as vacation or holiday schedule, break time, or work assignment (making sure it does not clash with seniority issues)

    e. professional development (for example, subscription to a journal or attendance or expenses for a professional conference)

    f. letters of recognition

    g. other (for example, preferred parking, theater tickets, gift certificates, flowers, food, or allow the employee to choose from a gift catalog)

REVIEW ACTIVITIES

Questions

1. An employee's daily performance to meet job requirements includes which of the following?

    a. being honest and trustworthy with patients and staff

    b. errors and incidents

    c. vacation time

    d. following policies and procedures when time allows

2. Specialized knowledge and judgment used to diagnose and treat human responses to health problems is classified as:

    a. technical skills

    b. partnership skills

    c. leadership skills

    d. clinical skills

3. A desired relationship between two parties seeking to work together toward a common goal is:

    a. leadership

    b. partnership

    c. evaluation

    d. promotion

4. Effective nurse managers do which of the following to meet staff, client, and market goals?

    a.   allow staff to manage their own productivity issues

    b.   tell team members what they need

    c.   delay training to decrease costs

    d.   set up and encourage mentoring relationships

5. A more experienced nurse who guides a less experienced employee is called a(n):

    a.   mentor

    b.   network

    c.   adult learner

    d.   assistive worker

6. An adult learner who likes to go back over the steps of a procedure and mentally review them would be using which adult learning stage?

    a.   experiencing

    b.   reflecting

    c.   relating

    d.   planning

7. According to the neuro-linguistic programming model of adult learning, a person who learns by reading an illustrated outline of a procedure is which type of learner?

    a.   visual

    b.   auditory

    c.   kinesthetic

    d.   intelligent

8. The abbreviation FTE means:

    a.   flex-time employment

    b.   full-time equivalent

    c.   first-time employee

    d.   full-time employment

9. The care delivery model in which one nurse is responsible for all aspects of patient care for that nurse's shift is called:

    a.   functional nursing

    b.   team nursing

    c.   total patient care

    d.   patient-focused care

10. Which of the following is a key activity for nurse managers who are evaluating staff performance?

    a.   avoid specifying specific behaviors, to provide latitude for employee creativity

    b.   enforce performance measurements and standards of care at all times

c. delegate feedback about goals and plans to other staff members
d. reinforce prior employee achievements to help employees find new
    ways to excel

Critical Thinking Questions

1. Choose a clinical care activity with which you are familiar (such as giving a bath, drawing blood, starting an IV, or other activity) and identify different ways to teach these activities to meet the needs of each of the four main types of adult learners.
2. Many health care organizations are using creative staffing approaches such as 10- and 12-hour shifts that give nurses additional days off during the week. Explain how to use the concept of FTEs to plan staffing when nurses work these long shifts.
3. For a nursing unit in which you work or have recently done a clinical rotation, describe the care delivery model. Is it effective, considering the staffing resources and patient acuity on the unit? If not, which model might work better?
4. Examine a few clinical pathways from different units in an organization in your community. Does the pathway include only nursing benchmarks, or is it multidisciplinary? Are pathways designed for surgical and medical diagnoses similar or different? What role does the patient play in meeting the pathway's outcomes?

Discussion Questions

1. In your nursing school, who is responsible for evaluating your performance? Is that person effective or ineffective? List the three aspects of your evaluation that are effective, and three that could be improved with suggestions for how they can be improved.
2. What evaluation method(s) does your workplace or school use to evaluate your performance? What are the advantages and disadvantages?
3. If you are responsible for evaluating employees or students, how do you evaluate their clinical, technical, and interpersonal skills?

Works Cited

Baker, C. M., Lamm, G. M., Winter, A. R., Robblecloth, V. B., Ransom, C. A., Conly, F., et al. (1997). Differentiated nursing practice: Assessing the state-of-the-science. *Nursing Economics, 15*(5), 253–261.

Bernat, A. L. (2003). Effective staffing. In P. Kelly-Heidenthal (Ed.), *Nursing leadership & management* (pp. 238–265). Clifton Park, NY: Thomson Delmar Learning.

Costello-Nickitas, D. (1997). *Quick reference to nursing leadership*. Clifton Park, NY: Thomson Delmar Learning.

Gardner, H. (1983). *Frames of mind: The theory of multiple intelligences*. New York: Basic Books.

Gouillart, F. J., & Sturdivant, B. (1994). Spend a day in the life of your customers. *Harvard Business Review, 72*, 25.

Lichtig, L. K., Knaug, R. A., Rison-McCoy, R., & Wozniak, L. M. (2000). *Nurse staffing and patient outcomes in the inpatient hospital setting*. Washington, DC: American Nurses Association.

Manthey, M. (1980). *The practice of primary nursing*. Boston: Blackwell Scientific.

Reynolds, L. (2002). Stand and deliver. . . different learning styles. *Training Journal* (October), 8–12.

Sullivan, E. J., & Decker, P. J. (2001). *Effective leadership and management in nursing* (5th ed.). Upper Saddle River, NJ: Prentice Hall.

Vance, C., & and Olson, R. (1991). Mentorship. In J. J. Fitzpatrick, R. L. Taunton, & A. K. Jacox (Eds.). *Annual review of nursing research*, (pp. 175–200). New York: Springer.

VanDerWall, S. (1998). Enhancing learning in training and adult education. *HRMagazine, 43*(7), 191.

Additional Resources

Atack, L. J. (2003). Becoming a web-based learner: Registered nurses' experiences. *Journal of Advanced Nursing, 44*(3), 289–297.

Bylone, M. (2004). Manage by mentoring. *Nursing Management, 35*(7), 6.

Byrne, M. W., & Keefe, M. (2002). Building research competence in nursing through mentoring. *Journal of Nursing Scholarship, 34*, 391–396.

Dix, G., & Hughes, S. J. (2004). Strategies to help students learn effectively. *Nursing Standard, 18*(32), 39–43.

Dobbin, K. R. (2001). Applying learning theories to develop teaching strategies for the critical care nurse: Don't limit yourself to the formal classroom lecture. *Critical Care Nursing Clinics of North America, 13*(1), 1–11.

Fahy, M. (2001). Assessing the quality of nursing performance. Teaching and assessing a new member of staff. *Assignment, 7*(3), 22–27.

Lander, J. (2004). The gift of mentoring. *Clinical Nursing Research, 13*(3), 175–179.

Measuring nursing care. (2004). *American Nurse, 36*(2), 6.

Milton, C. L. (2004). The ethics of personal integrity in leadership and mentorship: A nursing theoretical perspective. *Nursing Science Quarterly, 17*(2), 116–120.

Nursing performance measurement standards report. (2003). *MedNet, 9*(12), 12.

Simpson, R. L. (2004). Who's minding our profession? *Nursing Management, 35*(6), 13–15.

Spath, P. L. (2004). Practical guide for improving performance. *OR Manager, 20*(3), 23, 25–26.

Walsh, E. (2003). Get results with workload measurement. *Nursing Management* (IT Solutions Supplement), *34*(10), 16–18.

Web Sites

Hospital Nurse Staffing and Quality of Care: AHRQ
http://www.ahrq.gov/research/nursestaffing/nursestaff.htm

Managed Care Effect on Nursing Quality
http://www.sba.uconn.edu/healthcare/files/working-papers/2001-02.pdf

National Institute of Adult Continuing Education (NIACE)
http://www.niace.org.uk

National Quality Forum
http://www.qualityforum.org

Nurse Staffing, Models of Care Delivery and Interventions: AHRQ
http://www.ahrq.gov/research/nursestaffing/nursestaff.htm

Nurse Staffing and Patient Outcomes: HRSA Bureau of Health Professions
http://bhpr.hrsa.gov/nursing/staffstudy.htm

Principles for Nurse Staffing: American Nurses Association
http://www.nursingworld.org/readroom/stffprnc.htm

NURSES AS PROFESSIONAL LEADERS INSIDE AND OUTSIDE THE HEALTH CARE ORGANIZATION

CHAPTER 16

KEY TERMS

American Nurses Association
certification
expert speaker
informatics

professional nursing associations
publishing
self-education

KEY POINTS

1. Nursing leadership skills that can be used inside the health care organization

   A. **Publishing** (nurse to nurse publications)

      i. books
         a. research studies (for example, results of a hospital program to reduce postoperative infections for surgical patients; effects of a clinical pathway on length of stay)
         b. leadership/management issues (such as this book)
         c. clinical issues (for example, a review of the latest research and evidence-based practice concerning prevention of osteoporosis and how to translate research to practice)
         d. technical issues (for example, using a handheld informatics system to process and store essential patient information)
         e. textbooks (for example, on basic science and nursing, nursing process, anatomy and physiology, developing care plans, clinical delegation, emergency nursing, etc.)
         f. collections of work by other experts in a field or area (can be on any topic, and provide a range of views and expertise)
         g. time and effort requirement is high; authors receive royalties (money based on a percentage of sales); recognition and prestige are generally high

    ii. journals

- a. may be research based, clinical applications, specialty-based or general practice
- b. articles may be about practical applications, case studies, successes/failures, or reviews of the literature or editorials
- c. journals are usually peer reviewed; therefore, articles go through an extensive examination process with feedback provided to the author by other nurses
- d. case study reports are an ideal way to be published for first-time authors
- e. time and effort requirement, medium to high; authors are generally paid in copies, or sometimes a small stipend and do not receive royalties; recognition and prestige are generally high

   iii. newsletters

- a. often focus on practical articles for a specific nursing subgroup
- b. can be researched, written, and published in a relatively short time
- c. time and effort requirement, medium to low; authors may or may not be paid; recognition and prestige are lower than for journals and books

   iv. online

- a. anything that can be published on paper can also be published online (and increasingly, publications are electronic only)
- b. in addition, there are increasing numbers of Web-based tutorials that accompany textbooks, sites that act as information clearinghouses, sites that act as portals for continuing education, and commercial sites that sell products or information
- c. for example, the **American Nurses Association** publishes the *Online Journal of Issues in Nursing*, a scholarly journal available at no charge
- d. time and effort requirement varies, depending on the nature of the online work

B. **Professional nursing associations**

    i. these associations provide a number of services to nurses, including

- a. continuing education (both online and paper-based)
- b. job placement and job searches
- c. information clearinghouses
- d. advocacy and political action, not provided by all organizations, partly because of complex tax rules that set limits on the political activities of a professional organization. Some organizations establish political action committees (PAC) to separate the political work and lobbying from the organization's other work.

        e. professional publications and conferences

        f. sharing of information in general nursing practice or in a nursing specialty

        g. providing a community for nurses with similar interests; for example, the National League for Nurses focuses on nursing educators

    ii. many specialty nursing organizations provide services to nurses who work in a particular practice area, such as:

- American Academy of Ambulatory Care Nursing
- American Academy of Nurse Practitioners
- American Assembly for Men in Nursing
- American Association of Colleges of Nursing
- American Association of Critical-Care Nurses
- American Association of Legal Nurse Consultants
- American Association of Nurse Anesthetists
- American Association of Nurse Attorneys
- American College of Nurse-Midwives
- American Holistic Nurses Association
- American Organization of Nurse Executives
- American Psychiatric Nurses' Association
- American Society for Long-Term Care Nurses
- Association of Community Health Nursing
- Association of Nurses in AIDS Care
- Association of Operating Room Nurses
- Association of Rehabilitation Nurses
- Association of Women's Health, Obstetric, and Neonatal Nurses
- National Association of Neonatal Nurses
- National Black Nurses Association
- National Gerontological Nursing Association
- North American Nursing Diagnostics Association
- Transcultural Nursing Society
- Wound, Ostomy, and Continence Nurses Society

C. **Self-education.** Because health and nursing information is constantly changing, effective nurse leaders must be committed to being life-long learners. There are a number of ways by which nurses can meet this professional challenge.

    i. take responsibility for professional development; be proactive, constantly seek formal and informal learning opportunities; work with a mentor from whom you can learn whenever possible

    ii. achieve additional training, such as advanced cardiac life support (ACLS), neonatal resuscitation program (NRP), or pediatric advanced life support (PALS) and **certification,** such as board certification in a number of specialties through the American Nurses Credentialing Center, or through specialty organizations, such as

becoming a certified emergency nurse (CEN) or becoming certified in critical care nursing (CCRN), orthopedics (ONC), periop-
erative nursing (CNOR), or neuroscience nursing (CNRN), to
name but a few

   iii. keep up-to-date with developments in the field; professional journals are particularly helpful in this area

   iv. network with other nurses; tap the expertise of both—the people
inside the organization (through nursing or clinical practice committees, for example) or, learn from other practitioners outside
the organization (for example, by attending professional conferences where participants earn continuing education credits that
document attendance)

   v. learn about the business aspects of nursing and health care organizations, in addition to the clinical aspects

   vi. never say, "I know everything I need to know about my field."

   vii. learn and use **informatics** available; do not be a computer or
technology "avoider." Information systems that handle patient,
insurance, and organizational data are commonplace, and will
become more integrated into clinical practice in the future.

D. **Expert speakers** at nursing and other health care conventions

   i. most conventions actively seek knowledgeable, dynamic experts
who can motivate and inform listeners.

   ii. how to get started

     a. stake out your place as "expert"—learn something that not
many other people know; or use a special circumstance in the
organization or a case study of a complicated or unusual
patient situation to become the expert on that topic

     b. be aware of opportunities to teach others, such as caring for a
patient with an usual condition, or a unique combination of
factors that nurses manage successfully

     c. build and refine organizational skills to provide information
that is logical and understandable

     d. take a public speaking course, or call the local chapter of
Toastmasters International

     e. seek out a mentor who is a public speaker in nursing, and
ask for help to explore opportunities to learn how to speak
effectively, such as at small meetings within the organization,
or a local meeting of a nursing organization

     f. be aware of and able to use current presentation technology
(such as PowerPoint, LCD projectors, wireless microphones)

E. Continuing education for other professionals. Nurses are generally
effective at teaching patients, and they can transfer those teaching
skills to educate other professionals.

    i. other nurses
      a. inside the organization
      b. outside the organization, for example, professional confer-
         ences, or via continuing education material in written or mul-
         timedia formats
    ii. other health care staff, for example, phlebotomists, physical or
       occupational therapists, radiologic technicians, or pharmacy
       technicians

2. Nursing leadership skills that can be used outside the health care
organization

  A. Publishing (nurse to other professionals; materials for the public)

      i. books: for example, about health and safety tips, care during
        pregnancy, what to expect after surgery, etc
     ii. newsletters: especially newsletters geared to the general public,
        for example, about preventive care, specific health issues (for
        example, weight control, aging issues, women's issues)
    iii. journals: those for other health care professionals and magazines
        for the lay public
    iv. online: there are a growing number of online sites directed to the
        general public; most prefer authors with health care expertise;
        nurses who are able to write well are ideal candidates to produce
        these materials

  B. Professional associations other than nursing

      i. emergency nurses are ideal teachers for emergency medical tech-
        nicians and other emergency/rescue personnel through local or
        regional emergency services
     ii. organizations that provide education and services to the general
        public, such as local affiliates of the American Heart Association,
        the American Lung Association, or the American Red Cross
    iii. parish nurses, for example, provide comprehensive nursing care
        to members of a congregation in a faith-based setting
    iv. patient-focused groups, such as the National Emphysema and
        COPD Association welcome health care providers to work with
        patients to educate and empower them to manage their chronic
        health condition(s)

  C. Expert speakers at non-health care conventions

      i. local and regional health fairs for the community
     ii. providing a health care perspective for service organizations such
        as the Rotary, the Lions Club or parent-teacher associations
    iii. working with youth groups or scouting organizations

D.   Providing education for non-nursing professionals

   i.   teaching basic first aid
   ii. teaching CPR to community members and how to use an auto-
        mated external defibrillator (AED)
   iii. teaching camp counselors how to manage basic pediatric health
        issues

REVIEW ACTIVITIES

Questions

1. An article submitted to a peer-reviewed journal:
   a.   must have more than one author
   b.   is reviewed by other nurses
   c.   is reviewed by professional editors
   d.   must be a report on a research study

2. Which of the following publishing opportunities would take the least
   amount of time and effort?
   a.   writing a book
   b.   writing a journal article
   c.   writing a newsletter article
   d.   writing for a Web site

3. An ideal way for a nurse to publish his or her first article is by writing:
   a.   results of a clinical research study
   b.   a research review article
   c.   a case study report
   d.   a continuing education self-study article

4. The online journal published by the American Nurses Association is:
   a.   *Online Synthesis of Knowledge in Nursing*
   b.   *Online Study of Nursing Research*
   c.   *Online Journal of Nursing Knowledge*
   d.   *Online Journal of Issues in Nursing*

5. Which of the following is a service provided by all nursing associations?
   a.   sharing information among nurses with common interests
   b.   lobbying for a legislative agenda
   c.   certifying nurses in a specialty
   d.   publishing a national journal

6. This organization teaches people, public speaking skills:
   a. Toast of the Town
   b. Toastmasters International
   c. Toast to All Masters
   d. Toastmistress Association

7. A nurse can teach members of the community through:
   a. professional continuing education
   b. a local affiliate of the American Red Cross
   c. national nursing conventions
   d. articles in professional journals

Critical Thinking Questions

1. Review the three generalist nursing journals: *The American Journal of Nursing, Nursing 2006* (2007, etc) and *RN*. Are these journals peer-reviewed? How does a reader know if a journal is peer-reviewed? For each of these journals, identify an area in which a first-time author would have a good chance to be published.

2. Choose an area in which you would like more leadership experience: either writing or speaking. In the organization in which you work or have recently done a clinical rotation, find out if there is a nurse who has published an article or spoken at a local, regional or national meeting. Interview that nurse to learn how that nurse got his or her start in these leadership activities.

3. What opportunities are available in your community to teach? Is there a health fair at which you can do one-to-one teaching of community members? Does a health care organization hold classes for members of the community? How could you get involved in these programs?

Discussion Questions

1. What are the professional development activities or opportunities available to nurses at the organization where you work or do your clinical rotation? Describe activities both inside and outside the organization.

2. For two of the nursing associations listed on page 206, do a Web search and find the organization's home page. What activities does that organization engage in? Do they have a mission statement? What does that tell you about the organization and how it serves its members?

3. Setting aside your skills as a writer or public speaker, what topics would you be interested in writing or speaking about: (a) to other nurses; (b) to other health care professionals; (c) to the general public? What would be the most effective way to get this information to them (book, article, online, speaking)?

Works Cited

Costello-Nickitas, D. (1997). *Quick reference to nursing leadership.* Clifton Park, NY: Thomson Delmar Learning.

Jones, S. (2003). Emerging opportunities. In P. Kelly-Heidenthal (Ed.), *Nursing leadership & management* (pp. 532–549). Clifton Park, NY: Thomson Delmar Learning.

Additional Resources

American Nursing Association. (1994). *Standards for nursing professional development: Continuing education and staff development.* Washington, DC: Author.

Carroll, P. (2004). *What Nurses Know and Doctors Don't Have Time to Tell You.* New York: Perigee Books.

Cliff, B., & Martinez, J. (2004). Value of nursing certification. *Journal of Hospice and Palliative Nursing, 6*(3), 191–193.

Driscoll, J., & Driscoll, A. (2002). Writing an article for publication: An open invitation. *Journal of Orthopaedic Nursing, 6*(3), 144–152.

Farley, A. H. (2004). Be prepared: How to take the fear out of giving a presentation. *Professional Nurse, 19*(7), 410–412.

Gregg, M. M., & Pierce, L. L. (1994). Developing a paper for conference presentations. *Gastroenterology Nursing, 17*(1), 6–10.

Healy, P. (2004). Speak up for nursing. *Nursing Standard, 18*(33), 14–16.

Lundgren, J. (2004). To do in 2004: Get started on your publishing career. *ONS News, 19*(1), 14.

Payne, S. (2004). Conferences: Opportunities for all. *International Journal of Palliative Nursing, 10*(6), 268.

Smith, K., Bickford, C. J. (2004). Lifelong learning: Professional development, and informatics certification. *CIN: Computers, Informatics, Nursing, 22*(3), 172–178.

Starver, K. D. (2004). Professional presentations made simple. *Clinical Nurse Specialist, 18*(1), 16–20.

Web Sites

Note: This is a select list of nursing organizations and other sites. To find a specific organization, use a search engine such as google.com or yahoo.com.

American Nurses Association
    www.nursingworld.org

American Academy of Nurse Practitioners
www.aanp.org

American Assembly for Men in Nursing
www.aamn.org

American Association of Colleges of Nursing
www.aacn.nche.edu

American Association of Critical-Care Nurses
www.aacn.org

American Association of Legal Nurse Consultants
www.aalnc.org

American College of Nurse-Midwives
www.acnm.org

American Organization of Nurse Executives
www.aone.org

Association of Nurses in AIDS Care
www.anacnet.org

National Black Nurses Association
www.nbna.org

National League for Nursing: Self-education
www.nln.org/testprods/selfstudy.htm

North American Nursing Diagnostics Association
www.nanda.org

Transcultural Nursing Society
www.tcns.org

Toastmasters International
www.toastmasters.org

For a list of nurses' own Web sites, see Chapter 21.

Part IV

The Health Care Environment and its Impact on Nursing Leadership

17

CURRENT HEALTH CARE ENVIRONMENT (AND INTO THE FUTURE)

KEY TERMS

administration

capitation

diagnosis-related groups

framework

health care environment

health care environment trends

health maintenance organization

integrated health care systems

malpractice

Medicaid

Medicare

medicine

mentor

nursing

nursing trends

primary health care

prospective payment system

risk adjustment

secondary health care

tertiary health care

INTRODUCTION

The health care environment in the United States is complex and dynamic. It is affected by politics, culture and, of course, by the increasing competitiveness of the health care marketplace. Many changes that have occurred in recent years have been cost driven—an effort to provide high-quality patient outcomes, while keeping costs from rising. At the same time, many changes have resulted from nurses and other care providers implementing evidence-based care, standardizing practices across the care continuum, and providing as much equality of access and care as possible. Health care today is exciting and occasionally turbulent, with many opportunities for nurse leaders today and in the future.

KEY POINTS

1. Definition

    A.   The **health care environment** in the United States, according to Kelly-Heidenthal (2003), is complex and multifaceted

        i. it develops within a political environment that includes and is impacted by such concepts as:

           a. individualism

           b. civil liberties

           c. equality of process

           d. representative democracy

           e. capitalism and the belief in a free market economy

           f. concept of the separation of church and state (this concept is sometimes challenged by Catholic health systems, particularly with regard to reproductive health services; non-discrimination laws create ethical conflicts)

       ii. it is also impacted by the popular beliefs in a decentralized power structure and autonomy of action at the local levels of government and health care (Lockart, 1999)

      iii. as a result, health care systems in the United States

           a. have varying levels of care and differing amounts of resources

           b. provide cutting-edge, high technology interventions to some customers but not to others

           c. are not able to provide coordinated health care quality and access at a reasonable cost to all people

       iv. at present, many people in the United States (and the politicians who represent them) resist implementing a centralized, national health care system that would guarantee equal access and health coverage for all citizens, such as the health care programs in Canada and the United Kingdom

    B.   Health care can be categorized into three levels:

        i. **primary health care**

           a. goal is to promote health and prevent diseases by decreasing the risk to a person or a community

           b. this is accomplished through activities such as health education, immunization, lifestyle modification, referrals, and promoting a safe environment (for example, sanitation, workplace precautions, etc.)

           c. a challenge for the United States is the transition from a sickness model, in which primary care only addresses illness, to a wellness model, in which prevention and screening receive the same attention and funding as the current sickness model

  ii. **secondary health care**
   a. goal is to cure episodic, acute illnesses and use early and effective intervention to prevent disability or death
   b. this is accomplished through early detection and intervention; for example, using activities such as screenings, surgery, and acute medical care
  iii. **tertiary health care**
   a. goal is to minimize the effects of chronic or irreversible conditions/diseases
   b. this is accomplished through activities, such as education, providing direct care, and environmental modifications (Kelly-Heidenthal, 2003; Carroll, 2004)

C. The major types of health care organizations currently existing in the United States include:

  i. hospitals that are often characterized by length of stay and type of service
   a. acute care hospital: average stay is less than 30 days
   b. chronic care hospital: average length of stay is longer than 30 days (American Hospital Association, 1995)
   c. teaching hospital: hospital associated with a medical school that maintains house staff of residents on call and often also has students from a variety of health care disciplines
  ii. long-term care facilities
   a. provide skilled nursing services and occasionally rehabilitative services designed to foster self-care, but not goal-directed toward discharge
   b. nursing facilities provide daily nursing care
   c. residential care facilities provide a supportive environment for people who can no longer live independently, but no specialized care
  iii. subacute care facilities
   a. focus on rehabilitative care only
   b. length of stay is limited
   c. patients must show progress toward discharge goals
   d. increasingly used for patients whose care begins in an acute care hospital, but who no longer need the nurse: patient ratios in an acute care setting
   e. subacute care is much more cost-effective for stable patients than acute care
  iv. ambulatory care centers
   a. one of the fastest growing types of care
   b. includes physicians' offices, emergency rooms, outpatient surgery centers, special procedure centers, such as for

            endoscopy, diagnostic imaging centers, and family planning clinics

      c. most are free-standing and privately owned, but some are physically connected to acute-care hospitals and sometimes owned by those health care organizations

    v. home health care agencies

      a. intermittent, temporary delivery of health care to individuals in the home

      b. primary service provided is the nursing care for people recently discharged from hospital care to extend continuity of care

      c. may be provided by licensed or nonlicensed, skilled or non-skilled personnel

      d. may offer other professional services, such as physical or occupational therapy, durable medical equipment and other supplies

    vi. temporary service agencies

      a. provide nurses and other health care workers to hospitals that are short-staffed

      b. provide private duty nurses for individual patients

    vii. managed health care organizations

      a. a group of providers delivering services through an organized arrangement with a group of individuals

      b. managed health organizations are usually health maintenance organizations (HMOs), point of service organizations (POS), or preferred provider organizations (PPOs) (Sullivan & Decker, 2001)

D. The health care system in the United States consists of the following major groups of health professionals (Kelly-Heidenthal, 2003):

    i. **nursing:** including registered nurses, licensed practical (vocational) nurses, certified nurses aides, and a variety of assistive workers that operate under the direct supervision of a licensed nurse

    ii. other health professionals, such as respiratory therapists, physical therapists, social workers, and other clinical practitioners providing direct patient care or direct bedside care

    iii. **medicine:** physicians, either medical doctors (MD), osteopathic doctors (DO), or naturopathic physicians (NP), and dentists

    iv. **administration:** those involved in managing the "business" of health care

    v. increasingly, alternative medical providers are becoming the key members of the health care system, including chiropractic physicians, licensed massage therapists, and herbalists

E. Characteristics of the three major groups

    i. primary tasks and roles

    a. nursing: patient care; treating the human response to illness

    b. medicine: diagnosis and treatment of disease

    c. administration: providing system organization, management, continuity, and stability

  ii. demographics

    a. nursing: historically female, Caucasian, middle class; now increasing numbers of non-Caucasian nurses as well as men (although they remain the minority)

    b. medicine: historically white, middle to upper class male; in the last 5–7 years, however, roughly 50% of incoming medical school classes have been female

    c. administration: historically Caucasian male dominant; exception is Catholic hospitals, which have traditionally been run by Catholic sisters

  iii. perspective

    a. nursing: comforter, nurturer, educator; attending to the whole person, not just the disease; centered on patient

    b. medicine: diagnostician; greater emphasis on performing procedures; centered on treating and curing disease and the business aspects of running a practice

    c. administration: keeper of the status quo; protect against too much change or innovation; centered on the organization's business and market relationships; focus on allocation of resources

  iv. modes of conflict management

    a. nursing: interpersonal approach; get parties talking with one another; finding common ground

    b. medicine: maintaining hierarchy and control; use of authority and resources

    c. administration: structured, rational approach

  v. current major threats

    a. nursing: decrease in job security; constraints such as staffing levels, financial resources, human resources; changes in role from patient care to managing patient care through other personnel; aging workforce

    b. medicine: health economics; changing role in a managed care environment; loss of authority, income, and control of practice; professional accountability; malpractice suits and costs of malpractice insurance

    c. administration: decreased job security in managed care environment; organizational survival (Kelly-Heidenthal, 2003)

2. How health care is paid for

  A. Medicaid and Medicare

      i. created in 1965 by the Social Security Act, Title XVIII

     ii. **Medicaid** pays for health care services for people who are too poor to pay for care

   iii. **Medicare** pays for health care services for people who are aged 65 and over, or who are disabled or those with specified chronic health conditions

   iv. both systems originally used fee-for-service payment systems, reimbursing hospitals and physicians for the services delivered to patients

B.   Managed care

      i. Health Maintenance Organization Act was passed in 1973, in response to spiraling health care costs.

     ii. to fix costs, **health maintenance organizations** (HMOs) were given a fixed sum of money and were then responsible for delivering care to a specific group of patients for a preset fee, or **capitation**

   iii. checks were put in place to assure that quality was maintained while costs were reduced, such as

        a. peer-review organizations (PROs) focus on quality of care

   iv. other cost-reduction strategies

        a. development of diagnostic related groups (DRG) that allow for prospective payment by diagnosis; if an organization can provide care for less money than the established payment, there is a profit—if care costs more than the payment, there is a loss (see "C" below)

        b. limiting access to specialists by using primary care providers as gatekeepers; members can only receive reimbursement for specialist visits when approved by the primary care provider

        c. limiting expensive diagnostic tests

        d. providing financial incentives for physicians to cut costs in the form of bonuses when the organization reaches certain financial goals

        e. implementing clinical practice guidelines that are based on clinical research so as to standardize the most effective care for a variety of conditions and maximize efficiency

    v. because of consumer dissatisfaction with some HMO practices, many organizations have become more consumer oriented, with a focus on customer satisfaction as well as cost containment

C.   Prospective payment system

      i. implemented with the Tax Equity and Fiscal Responsibility (TEFRA) Act of 1982

     ii. TEFRA put a ceiling on Medicare payments for hospital services to control costs

   iii. it also led the way for amendments (1983) that mandated a **prospective payment system** (PPS)
   iv. PPS established **diagnosis-related groups** (DRGs), which
      a. provide payment based on the diagnosis
      b. force hospitals to provide care at a lower cost since reimbursement is less than under the fee-for-service model
      c. have led to a movement to standardize care, to maximize efficiency, and to reduce length of hospital stays

D. Impact of Balanced Budget Act of 1997

   i. provided comprehensive reform of Medicare, including
      a. expansion of Medicare's health plan offerings
      b. changes in how plans are paid by the government
      c. extension of PPS to ambulatory and post-acute care organizations
      d. strengthening of fraud and abuse regulations to stop payment for services not provided (Simms, Price, & Ervin, 2000)
   ii. designated nurse practitioners as fully qualified providers of all Part B services, with reimbursement at 85% of physicians' fee schedules (Kelly-Heidenthal, 2003)

3. Current trends in the health care environment. According to Sullivan and Decker (2001), current **health care environment trends** include:

A. Health care run by business people focused on cost-effectiveness

   i. in addition to legislation and government actions, marketplace changes are changing the way health care organizations operate
   ii. competition continues to force hospitals, physicians, and home care agencies to merge, join networks (often comprised of members providing different levels of care, such as acute care hospitals with subacute care facilities, long-term care and visiting nurse associations) and form integrated health care systems
   iii. **integrated health care systems** are organizations that deliver a continuum of care by providing coverage to a group of individuals, and accepting fixed payments for that group. They have emerged as organizations struggle to find ways to survive financially in the current competitive environment.
   iv. in integrated health care systems, the focus is on primary and preventive care as well as
      a. providing whole continuum of care; for example: from acute care hospitalization for a hip replacement to subacute care for rehabilitative services to home care to help patients modify the home environment as necessary
      b. providing geographic coverage

    c. accepting the risk of covering one group for a fixed payment

    d. moving toward health care systems rather than independently functioning health care entities

B. Multihospital systems, including international organizations

    i. complex legal arrangements that spread litigation cost and risk

    ii. rationing or controlling access to health care to control costs

    iii. decentralized systems that share human and financial resources, as well as technology (Sullivan & Decker, 1992)

C. Other cost-driven changes include:

    i. increased technological capabilities to prevent errors, such as computerized order-entry systems to eliminate potential errors associated with poor handwriting; streamline administrative functions, such as patient charges; control inventory, so that less storage space is required on-site with fewer dollars tied up in stock; and allow nurses to spend more time on patient care or management issues, rather than paperwork

    ii. outsourcing services to non-hospital/non-institutional providers; for example, laboratory services, radiology services, physical therapy services, and patient account management

    iii. increased number of complex ethical issues, including limiting services, such as transplants to people who have the means to pay; exploring whether expensive technological interventions and sophisticated critical care saves lives or prolongs deaths; and proper provision of end-of-life care, particularly pain management

    iv. patient teaching as major hospital "product" line. Although teaching has traditionally been a part of the nurse's job, hospitals are increasingly seeing the education component as a revenue-generating service, such as with certified diabetes educators and a diabetes education service or product line.

    v. integrated delivery systems

        a. horizontal: arrangements between or among organizations that provide the same or similar services to reduce duplication; for example, Main Street Hospital provides a dietician and a "healthy eating" program to Oak Lane Hospital, and Oak Lane Hospital provides mobile diagnostic radiology services (a portable mammography center) to Main Street Hospital

        b. vertical: an arrangement between or among dissimilar but related organizations to provide a continuum of services; for example, a home care nursing service affiliating with an acute care hospital to provide seamless post-discharge follow-up care. Vertical integration improves service coordination, is cost effective, promotes continuity of care, and uses human resources more efficiently (Newhouse & Mills, 1999; Sullivan & Decker, 2001).

   vi. Focus on preventive care

      a. population-based health care: based on preserving and improving the health of groups of people (community nursing or public health focus instead of home care, which focuses on individuals)

      b. disease management: using preventive care, environmental intervention, and lifestyle changes to prevent disease or decrease the effects of disease on a population or individual (Carroll, 2004)

4. According to Sullivan and Decker (1992), the following **nursing trends** are expected to continue into the near future:

  A. Increased corporate roles for nurses

     i. separate, third-party reimbursement for nursing services
     ii. nursing as major revenue producer, as nursing services become reimbursable

  B. Demand for nurses exceeds supply

     i. as the nursing shortage continues, nurses will have increasing responsibility, increased management roles, and a greater say in how care is managed and provided
     ii. nurses, especially RNs, will have greater advantage concerning pay, working conditions, benefits

  C. Joint practice: physicians and nurses

     i. number of advanced practice nurses and nurse practitioners will continue to grow
     ii. in many areas, there will be an increasing number of physician/nurse practitioner partnerships for providing care
     iii. nurse practitioners become primary care providers for underserved areas— often in rural and poor urban areas

  D. Working conditions

     i. RN's patient loads will continue to increase
     ii. a decrease in number of RNs (more patients per RN) will result in an increased use of LPN and other supportive personnel such as noncredentialed assistive workers (see "delegation" in Chapter 20)
     iii. this scenario has led to an increasingly entrepreneurial element in nursing, and this trend is expected to continue (see Chapter 21 on entrepreneurial opportunities)

E.   Role of Joint Commission on Accreditation of Healthcare Organizations (JCAHO) in current health care environment

   i.   JCAHO accreditation needed for hospitals to receive Medicare and Medicaid reimbursement
   ii.   all hospitals and other health care organizations that seek JCAHO accreditation must monitor patient outcomes and use a performance measurement system that provides data about outcomes and other care indicators
   iii.   most health care organizations agree on the need to standardize definitions as well as adjust data for severity of patient illness on admission (Kelly-Heidenthal, 2003)

F.   Patient outcomes and evidence based care. A number of variables affect patient outcomes (such as patient illness severity, noted above. See also Chapter 14)

   i.   **risk adjustment** is used to adjust patient data statistically to reflect significant patient variables
       a.   adjusts data for severity of patient illness
       b.   providers must still strive to create definitions and measurements that are consistent across all organizations, so that data can be accurately compared
   ii.   role of Agency for Healthcare Research and Quality (AHRQ)
       a.   formed in 1989 as part of the U.S. Public Health Service
       b.   was begun to develop clinical practice guidelines using the best available evidence
       c.   AHRQ also supports research into the effect of medical practices and has recently introduced a Web site dedicated to sharing information about medical errors [http://www.webmm.ahrq.gov] (McCormick, Cummings, & Kovner, 1997)

G.   Impact of **malpractice** concerns and care that does not meet acceptable standards of practice on current health care environment

   i.   Institute of Medicine reports
       a.   concluded that more people die from medication mistakes than from "highway accidents, breast cancer, or AIDS" (Kohn, Corrigan, & Donaldson, 1999)
       b.   identified information technology, payment, clinical knowledge, and the professional workforce as health care areas to target for future change to improve quality and reduce errors (Kohn, Corrigan, & Donaldson, 2001)
   ii.   JCAHO patient safety standards
       a.   accredited hospitals must implement an organization-wide safety program
       b.   hospitals must inform patients when care results differ significantly from anticipated outcomes (Lovern, 2001)

c. hospitals are required to report situations that resulted or could have resulted in patient death or serious injury (called sentinel events) so that situations can be analyzed and shared with other accredited organizations to prevent similar situations from occurring.

5. Basic **framework** for quality health care. According to Donabedian (1996), three conceptual areas make up a framework for quality health care.

   A.   Structure elements

      i.   lay a foundation for quality health care
      ii. identify structures that must be in place for a system to deliver quality care
      iii. for example, a well-constructed hospital, quality patient-care standards, effective staffing policies, and appropriate environmental standards

   B.   Process elements

      i.   build on structure elements
      ii. identify what nursing and health care interventions must be in place to deliver quality care
      iii. for example, management of health care process, and using clinical practice guidelines and nursing standards

   C.   Outcome elements

      i.   the end results of quality care
      ii. reflect the presence of structure and process elements
      iii. for example, one outcome, such as improvement of patient health, requires a quality hospital (structure) and quality treatment standards (process) (Kelly-Heidenthal, 2003)

6. Additional external forces that influence health care, and their implications for nurse leaders

   A.   Technological

      i.   technological advances
         a. expansion of treatment sites away from hospitals into ambulatory and mobile centers that better serve the needs of the community
         b. new treatment modalities and care sites needed to accommodate them; for example, freestanding surgical centers, chemotherapy centers, etc
         c. ongoing need for continuing education about and training for new systems

ii. information technology
    a. increased use of paperless environments
    b. central storage of patient information (often from multiple sites)
    c. increased use of handheld technology to access patient information, such as communication technologies
    d. confidentiality issues (see HIPAA, below)
    e. ongoing need for continuing education about and training for new systems

B. Population changes

   i. aging population
    a. increased demand for health care for people aged 65 to 75 years as this segment of the population grows
    b. increased demand for chronic care management for people aged 75 years and over
    c. ethical issues surrounding prolonging life, quality of life, and end of life care
   ii. increased diversity of population
    a. understanding and meeting variety of patient expectations by enhancing understanding of cultural diversity
    b. meeting the varied needs and understanding the different backgrounds of a multicultural work force
   iii. social morbidity, such as AIDS, drug abuse, violence
    a. dealing effectively with increases in demand for services
    b. compensating for shortages in some health care professional categories (for example, nursing, physical therapy, pharmacy)
    c. need to develop caregiver teams that can function across multiple treatment sites such as nurse-social worker teams

C. Globalization

   i. managing cross-national and cross-cultural referrals
   ii. increasing the competitiveness and productivity of U.S. labor force
   iii. managing alliances, especially biotechnology and new technology development (Kelly-Heidenthal, 2003)

D. Possibility of mass catastrophe due to terrorism

   i. biological, nuclear, chemical, incendiary, or explosive weapons
   ii. need for health care provider education and training and community readiness for public safety and first responders
   iii. need for health care consumer education (Carroll, 2004)

7. Recent changes in health care

A. Health Insurance Portability and Accountability Act (HIPAA)

       i. includes measures to standardize and computerize health care billing, claims transactions, processing, and reimbursement, including
         a. patients can review and request amendments to their medical records
         b. consumers have control over how their personal health information is used and limits the release of patient information without the patient's consent
         c. requires privacy-conscious business practices, such as training employees about patient confidentiality
         d. requires paper records and oral communication to be protected from breaches of privacy, such as not using postcards to remind patients to make appointments—using paper in a sealed envelope instead
      ii. requires patient data to be transferred securely and confidentially
     iii. this has meant significant changes in administrative operations and information services for most providers (Morrissey, 2001; Kelly-Heidenthal, 2003)

B. Public information about health plan quality (Medicare and Medicaid quality ranking)

       i. ranks states from best to work in terms of quality of care for the entire Medicare or Medicaid population treated
      ii. publishes and distributes information throughout the United States
     iii. based on this information, a "100 Top Hospitals" list is published each year (Kelly-Heidenthal, 2003)

C. PEW Health Professions Commission

       i. published reports on competencies, identifying 21 competencies that care providers need in order to give quality care in the 21st century
      ii. report calls for changes in institutions training nurses, physicians, and other health care personnel (O'Neil, 1998)
         a. develop programs to enhance diversity in education to better meet the needs of a diverse population
         b. reach out to K-12 schools to encourage students to enter the health professions
         c. incorporate public service into all educational programs for health professionals
         d. relocate training out of the institution and into the community

8. Current trends affecting the nursing role

A. Transdisciplinary nursing

    i. future health needs require a professional nurse who demonstrates caring, competence, and practice

    ii. transdisciplinary nursing focuses on the team of care providers, who bring various kinds of expertise to a team

    iii. more emphasis on a team and less emphasis on the team requiring a leader

    iv. with this model, patients and family have immediate access to any member of the team; there is no gatekeeper, and everyone on the team is responsible and accountable (Kelly-Heidenthal, 2003)

B. The role of the nursing mentor

    i. a **mentor** is "a wiser and more experienced person who guides, supports, and nurtures a less experienced person" (Sullivan & Decker, 1999, p. 505)

    ii. what mentors can do

      a. provide a present orientation—what needs to be done today, and how

      b. increase trust, confidence, and competence in the person being mentored

      c. increase the mentored person's self-esteem and job satisfaction

    iii. how to develop a mentor relationship

      a. look for senior team members and ask for advice

      b. look for someone who has already been a mentor

      c. choose more than one mentor to develop different skills; for example, one mentor in clinical practice and one in professional development

      d. do not expect the mentor relationship to provide all needs

      e. the nurse needs to maintain his or her responsibility by not exploiting the relationship with the mentor or wasting the mentor's time (Sullivan & Decker, 1992)

REVIEW ACTIVITIES

Questions

1. Which of the following has a significant impact on health care in the United States?

    a. increased resources to fund health care

    b. strong Federal government control over local decisions

    c. aging of the population and longer life expectancy

    d. integrated health care services

2. The goal of primary health care is to:
   a. control access to services
   b. promote health and prevent diseases
   c. cure episodic, acute diseases
   d. minimize the effects of chronic disease

3. Which of the following health care entities provides care to acutely ill patients for less than 30 days?
   a. subacute care facility
   b. hospital
   c. skilled nursing facility
   d. ambulatory care center

4. Which of the following statements is true about home care organizations?
   a. they focus on the care of populations, not individuals
   b. they may offer professional services as well as durable medical equipment
   c. they can provide care only by licensed personnel
   d. they provide permanent, ongoing health care services to a community

5. The group of health care professionals that is associated with the business of providing health care is:
   a. nursing
   b. medical
   c. allied health
   d. administrative

6. The program that provides for health care services for disabled persons is:
   a. Medicare
   b. Medicaid
   c. DRGs
   d. PPS

7. Capitation is defined as:
   a. preset fee for delivering care to a specific group of people
   b. payment based on the diagnosis a patient receives
   c. designation of nurse practitioners as fully qualified providers under Part B of Medicare
   d. the information-sharing limits imposed by HIPAA

8. An arrangement made between or among organizations that provide the same or similar services is called:
   a. horizontal integrated delivery system
   b. fee for service system
   c. population-based care system
   d. joint practice delivery system

9. The entity that oversees whether health care organizations meet standards that keep them eligible for Medicare and Medicaid reimbursement is:
   a. Agency for Healthcare Research and Quality
   b. Joint Commission on Accreditation of Healthcare Organizations
   c. Health Insurance Portability and Accountability Act
   d. Pew Health Professions Commission

10. Which of the following is a characteristic of a mentor?
   a. a health professional from a different field or specialty area
   b. an experienced member of a health care team who shares expertise with less experienced colleagues
   c. a person who supplies all the needs of a subordinate staff member
   d. a person who is responsible for orientation of new employees

Critical Thinking Questions

1. A nurse working in a Catholic hospital that is the only source of health care in a poor inner-city neighborhood learns from a patient that the hospital prohibits tubal ligations and vasectomies. The nurse is concerned that members of the community cannot receive a full range of legal health-related services. Describe how this nurse should approach this ethical dilemma.

2. What are the top 5 DRGs in the organization in which you work or in which you have done a clinical rotation? How do those diagnostic related groups correlate to the demographics of the population served by the organization? (For demographic data, visit http://www.census.gov).

3. What is the closest subacute care facility in your area? How is this facility different from the acute care hospital(s)? Examine issues, such as the common diagnoses, nurse to patient ratio, staff mix, and presence or absence of other health professionals in the organization.

Discussion Questions

1. How has managed care affected the health care which you and your family receive and the environment in which you work, or have your clinical experience? Name as many examples as you can think of.

2. Do you think these managed care impacts are primarily positive or negative? Why? Give examples.

3. Which nursing trends do you see as the most positive for your future practice as a professional registered nurse? Which ones concern you most? Why?

4. Based on your experience, name the qualities of an effective mentor. Describe a positive experience you have had with a mentor, and identify an area in which you would like to have a mentor.

Works Cited

American Hospital Association (1995). *AHA guide to the health care field*. Chicago: Author.

Carroll, P. (2004). *Community health nursing: A practical guide*. Clifton Park, NY: Thomson Delmar Learning.

Donabedian, A. (1996). Evaluating the quality of medical care. *Milbank Memorial Fund Quarterly, 44*, 194–196.

Kelly-Heidenthal, P. (2003). America's health care environment. In P. Kelly-Heidenthal, *Nursing Leadership & Management* (pp. 1–31). Clifton Park, NY: Thomson Delmar Learning.

Kohn, L., Corrigan, J., & Donaldson, M. (Eds.) (1999). *To err is human: Building a safer health system.* Committee on Quality of Care in America, Institute of Medicine. Washington, DC: National Academy Press.

Kohn, L., Corrigan, J., & Donaldson, M. (Eds.) (2001). *Crossing the quality chasm: A new health system for the 21st century.* Committee on Quality of Care in America, Institute of Medicine. Washington, DC: National Academy Press.

Lockart, C. A. (1999). Health care delivery in the United States. In J. E. Hitchcock, P. E. Schubert, & S. A. Thomas, *Community health nursing*. Clifton Park, NY: Thomson Delmar Learning.

Lovern, E. (2001). JCAHO's new tell-all. Standards require that patients know about below-par care. *Modern Healthcare, 31*(1), 2, 15.

McCormick, K. A., Cummings, M. A., & Kovner, C. (1997). The role of the Agency for Health Care Policy and Research in improving outcomes of care. *Nursing Clinics of North America, 32*(3), 5.

Morrissey, J. (2001). Slow down: HIPAA ahead. *Modern Healthcare*, 30.

Newhouse, R. P., & Mills, M. E. (1999). Vertical systems integration. *Journal of Nursing Administration, 29*(10), 22–29.

O'Neil, E. H., and the Pew Professions Commission. (December 1998). *Recreating health professional practice for a new century*. San Francisco: Pew Health Professions Commission.

Simms, L. M., Price, S. A., & Ervin, N. E. (2000). *Professional practice of nursing administration* (3rd ed.). Clifton Park, NY: Thomson Delmar Learning.

Sullivan, E. J., Decker, P. J. (1992). *Effective management in nursing* (3rd ed.). Redwood City, CA: Addison-Wesley Publishing.

Sullivan, E. J., Decker, P. J. (2001). *Effective leadership and management in nursing* (5th ed.). Upper Saddle River, NJ: Prentice Hall.

Additional Resources

Brous, E. A. (June 2004). 7 tips on avoiding malpractice claims. *Nursing*, 34, 16–19.

Carroll, P. *The Surgical Nurses' Managed Care Manual* (1999). Boston, MA: Total Learning Concepts

Feagin, J. R. & McKinney, K. D. (2003). *The many costs of racism*. Lanham, MD: Rowman & Littlefield.

Foldy, S. L., et al. (2004). The public health dashboard: A surveillance model for bioterrorism preparedness. *Journal of Public Health Management & Practice, 10*(3), 234–242.

Haas-Wilson, D. (2003). *Managed care and monopoly power: The antitrust challenge.* Cambridge, MA: Harvard University Press.

JCAHO to Shift to Unannounced Surveys by 2006. (2004). *Urologic Nursing, 24*(3), 228.

Christiansen, D. A. (2004). Medication management: Saving lives one order at a time. *Nursing* Management, *16*(5), 16.

Jennings, C. P. (2004). Living with change and meeting the challenge. *Policy, Politics & Nursing Practice, 5*(3), 143–145.

Karch, A. M. (2004). Practice errors. What's wrong with U? JCAHO places limits on abbreviations used in practice. *American Journal of Nursing, 104*(6), 65–66.

Lander, J. (2004). The gift of mentoring. *Clinical Nursing Research, 13*(3), 175–179.

Mentoring the minority nurse leader of tomorrow. (2004). *Nursing Administration Quarterly, 28*(3), 165–170.

New JCAHO documentation guidelines required nationwide. (February 2004). *Nursing, 34,* 2.

Povar, G. J., et al. (2004). Ethics in practice: Managed care and the changing health care environment. *Annals of Internal Medicine, 140*(4), 131–138.

Robinson, D., & Kish, C. P. (Eds.) (2001). *Core concepts in advanced practice nursing.* St. Louis, MO: Mosby.

Web Sites

American Hospital Association
   http://www.aha.org

AHA: HIPAA Home Page
   http://www.hospitalconnect.com/aha/key_issues/hipaa

AHRQ
   http://www.ahrq.gov

AHRQ morbidity and mortality information
   http://www.webmm.ahrq.gov

Centers for Medicare and Medicaid Services
http://www.cms.hhs.gov/

e-Health Internet Code of Ethics
http://www.ihealthcoalition.org

Health care spending statistics
http://www.hcfa.gov/stats/nhe-oact/tables/chart.htm

HIPAA
http://www.hipaa.org
http://www.cms.hhs.gov/HIPAAGanInfo/

JCAHO
www.jcaho.org

National Center for Health Statistics
http://www.cdc.gov/nchs

National Coalition on Health Care
http://www.nchc.org

NURSING LEADERS INFLUENCING POLITICS AND ACTING AS PATIENT ADVOCATES

CHAPTER 18

KEY TERMS

demographics

empowerment

minority populations

partnerships

patient advocacy

political arenas

political lobbies

politics

INTRODUCTION

The general public may be cynical about "politics"—whether it is the political process in which we elect officials to serve in the government, or whether the term is used to describe the unofficial power structure in an organization. However, politics has a significant impact on organizations in general and health care organizations in particular. Nurses have always been advocates for patient care. Nurses who are politically savvy can advocate not only for individual patients, but also for organizations, communities, and entire populations. This chapter discusses the role of the nurse advocate/politician.

KEY POINTS

1. Trends in U.S. health care and nursing roles

    A.   Politics and economics of human services

        i. **politics**
          a. a "process by which people use a variety of methods to achieve their goals" (Miller, 2003, p. 141)
          b. politics exist because resources are limited and some people have more resources than others

    ii. politics is not a dirty word in health care
- a. nurses who can effectively compete, negotiate, and collaborate with others to get what they need have strong political skills
- b. these nurses can build strong bases of support for themselves, their organization, and for the overall nursing profession (Miller, 2003)

    iii. a variety of **political arenas** exist
- a. in the workplace, to advocate for nursing within the organization
- b. in the government, to influence who gets what kind of health care, when, where and how
- c. in financing, to influence where patients receive care and how care and resources are financed and allocated
- d. in the organization, to influence the kind of care a patient receives, based on the organization's policies and procedures
- e. in the community, to influence public/community health, or to advocate for underserved populations (Sullivan & Decker, 2001)

    iv. the benefits of a politically savvy nurse
- a. political **empowerment** means a better chance of getting a share of, or controlling the distribution of, resources
- b. understands that health care consumers are also a political organization that must be dealt with effectively

    v. the role of **minority populations**
- a. the United States has about 80 million racially and ethnically diverse people (Leddy & Pepper, 1998)
- b. people from different cultures and backgrounds have different ways of promoting health, different ideas about illness and behavior, respond differently to illness, and have different ideas about the role of health care providers
- c. nurses who understand and value diversity can form political partnerships with consumer groups of various ethnic or cultural backgrounds to promote common health care goals

    vi. the role of changing **demographics,** especially age
- a. the aging population will be the most rapidly growing demographic in the United States, due to the "baby boom" generation, born between 1946 and 1964
- b. on January 1, 2008, the first members of the baby boom will be able to apply for Social Security benefits
- c. this population is affecting health care at every level
- d. this age group is particularly vocal about entitlements such as Social Security and Medicare
- e. many in this group are members of powerful **political lobbies** and organizations that advance their interests and concerns such as the AARP (Miller, 2003)

B. Nurses and **patient advocacy**

    i. the nursing role is one of patient advocate

    ii. nurses have traditionally provided hands-on care

        a. in the process, nurses learn about patients and know their needs

        b. nurses act as advocates and liaisons between the patient and the doctor, family and doctor, or patient/family and the health care system

    iii. the current health care climate has made this role more problematic; some critics cite an eroding of the advocacy role of the nurse (O'Connell, 2000)

C. The nurse as political advocate and activist

    i. understanding organizations and political strategies

        a. health policies affect both nurses and consumers (and nurses as consumer of health care services)

        b. consumers may not know that nurses can be political forces as well as patient care advocates

    ii. the politics of health issues and funding

        a. nurses can form partnerships with consumer groups

        b. coalitions have more political power and a stronger political voice, as well as a variety of expertise (Miller, 2003)

    iii. traditional electoral politics

        a. the 2004 presidential race established nurses as an important constituency group started by *Nurses4Dean*, a national group of nurse leaders supporting the candidacy of Howard Dean, M.D., established in early 2003

        b. in 2004, organizations such as "Nurses for Kerry" and "Nurses for Bush" were formally established with their own Web sites and political action strategies

        c. these organizations are important because they were formed from the grassroots by nurse leaders who had a unique perspective on health care issues; these groups were not established by organized labor or through endorsements of national nursing organizations such as the ANA

        d. the 108th Congress had three nurse members along with eight physicians, three dentists, an optometrist, and a pharmacist (Amer, 2004)

D. Consumer-oriented advocacy

    i. consumers' need for accountability

        a. consumers paying higher portion of health care costs out-of-pocket

        b. as a result, consumers are demanding more accountability and information

      ii. nurses can also work to
- a. increase patients' rights
- b. provide political vision and insight to help make the health care system more patient-focused
- c. advocate for the best care for the greatest possible number of people.

2. Skills required to establish **partnerships** with consumer groups

A.   Preliminary work

     i. listen
- a. be sensitive to health care needs
- b. understand the political nature of the potential consumer/ partner
- c. see concerns from the consumer's point of view

     ii. study
- a. seek out representative and opposing consumer viewpoints
- b. use consumer group meetings, focus groups, literature, and interviews to gather information

    iii. assess
- a. determine need, value, and context of partnership
- b. establish boundaries of the partnership

    iv. focus
- a. identify, along with consumer group, the purpose of the partnership
- b. articulate goals and specific objectives

     v. compromise and negotiate
- a. work through nonessential/noncritical points.
- b. agree on partnership's position and responsibilities

    vi. plan
- a. develop a political strategy
- b. objective to achieve designated partnership goals

   vii. test and model
- a. test the political waters and get feedback on the plan from key stakeholders and other involved parties
- b. model the political work and define the structure for working with other partners

B.   Once partnership is established

     i. direct political action
- a. understand the big picture
- b. clearly define what situations are amenable to change and which are not, and do not waste time and resources on those that cannot be changed; concentrate on what can be changed

      ii. implement action
         a. align political support
         b. take action
     iii. network and build political credibility
         a. assemble an adequate base of support in terms of money, people, and time
         b. participate in policy-making efforts that support the partnership and its agenda
     iv. bargain
         a. downplay rivalries
         b. address conflict in a timely and constructive manner
      v. report, publicize, and lobby
         a. get the partnership's message to the public
         b. draw attention to the needs of the consumer group
         c. establish relationships with elected officials and other people of influence who can lend credibility and be change agents

C.   Follow up: regularly evaluate work and proceed as needed (Miller, 2003)

3. Ways of acting as a nurse advocate and leader

A.   Lobbying at local and national levels

      i. for health care regulations
      ii. for guidelines that serve a consumer group's interest

B.   Consulting with representatives from consumer groups when health legislation is being written

C.   Monitoring health care legislation and its enforcement

      i. becoming involved in a watchdog agency to protect consumer rights
      ii. ensuring that punitive or corrective action occurs when health care legislation is not enforced or followed
      ii. providing feedback to elected officials about how legislation may need to be amended once it has been implemented and problems identified

D.   Encouraging providers and payors

      i. to make changes in service delivery and to continually review for quality and customer satisfaction
      ii. to voluntarily meet changing consumer demands

E.   Educating consumers and lawmakers

      i. develop and distribute materials
      ii. work to change perceptions of consumers, legislators, or people in the media as needed

F.   How to maintain credibility in politics

    i.   nurses must demonstrate
      a.   professional competence
      b.   professional accountability that exceeds consumer expectations
    ii.   ways to assert professional credibility
      a.   become lifelong learners and demonstrate continuous professional growth
      b.   approach nursing as a service to the public
      c.   take ownership of situations
      d.   work to resolve problems and overcome obstacles to providing care (Miller, 2003)

G.   Impact of politics on nurses' futures

    i.   nurses know the health care system's problems
    ii.   nurses also have many of the solutions
    iii.   nursing input into health care policy is no longer an option—it is a necessity
    iv.   future nurses need to be prepared to demand a seat at the policy-making table (at any level—local, state, national)

REVIEW ACTIVITIES

Questions

1.   A process by which people use a variety of methods to achieve their goals is called:

    a.   empowerment
    b.   demographics
    c.   patient advocacy
    d.   politics

2.   The political arena that nurses may operate in to influence public health or advocate for underserved populations is:

    a.   the workplace
    b.   health care financing
    c.   the community
    d.   the government

3.   This gives people a better chance of getting a share of, or control of distribution of, resources:

    a.   empowerment
    b.   patient advocacy

    c. accountability

    d. political vision

4. In forming partnerships with consumer groups, a nurse advocate who uses consumer group meetings, focus groups, literature, and interviews is using which of the following skills?

    a. compromising

    b. test/modeling

    c. studying

    d. implementation

5. Which of the following is a way of acting as a nurse leader and advocate?

    a. lobby only at the national level so as to achieve the greatest influence

    b. encourage payors and providers to make changes in service delivery

    c. avoid punitive action when legislation is not enforced

    d. educate consumers to follow the policies of third-party payors

Critical Thinking Questions

1. For the first time, in the 2004 presidential campaign, there were coalitions of nurses involved in the campaigns: *Nurses for Bush* and *Nurses for Kerry*. Do a search on the Internet to see if the Web sites still exist. Compare the goals of each group. How are these groups different from nursing organizations such as the ANA that endorse political candidates?

2. Why is it that some nursing organizations endorse candidates (ANA) and others do not (American Association of Critical-Care Nurses, Emergency Nurses Association)? How do you feel about a national nursing organization that endorses a candidate for president of the United States? Is that an appropriate role for a nursing organization? Why or why not? Does a nursing organization whose endorsed candidate loses lose power in the political arena?

3. Which nursing organization(s) in your state monitor(s) legislation on the state level? What is the role of the state board of nursing in the legislative process? Learn what legislative initiatives are planned for the current or upcoming session of your legislature for health care in general or nursing, in particular. What are the pros and cons? Who supports the legislation and who opposes it?

4. Choose a bill under consideration in your state legislature and decide whether you think your representative should vote for it or against it. Make an appointment to meet with your representative to share your concerns and urge your representative to vote as you would.

5. All members of Congress have local offices in which they meet the constituents so that they do not have to travel to Washington, D.C. Choose an

area about which you feel strongly, such as reducing cost of prescription drugs for seniors, funding of scholarships for nursing education, or establishing community health care centers, for example. Check with local and national nursing organizations to learn about the bills that will be considered by Congress, and those on which your representative will vote. Develop five bullet points that support your position on one of these issues and then make an appointment to meet with your member of Congress to share your concerns.

6. Visit the website http://www.nationalnurse.org what is the concept of a National Nurse? Is this a good idea? Why or why not?

Discussion Questions

1. What political activities (nursing or otherwise) have you been involved in? Was your experience a positive or negative one? Why? What did you learn to make your experience more productive the next time?

2. What nursing advocacy activities are available at your workplace? How would you become involved?

3. Based on your experience, what would be the most important skills for a nurse activist/advocate to have? In your area, how could a nurse acquire those skills?

4. In your community or in your state, does a nurse hold elected office? If so, invite him or her to speak to your class about how they got involved in the political process and how they see their background as a nurse contributing to their role in elected office.

5. Are you registered to vote? If not, why not? List three ways people in your community can register to vote in the next election.

Works Cited

Amer, M.L. (2004 October 25). *Membership of the 108th Congress: A Profile.* CRS Report for Congress. Available at: http://www.senate.gov/reference/resources/pdf/RS21379.pdf.

Leddy, S., & Pepper, J. M. (1998). *Conceptual bases of professional nursing* (4th ed.). Philadelphia: Lippincott.

Miller. T. (2003). Politics and consumer partnerships. In P. Kelly-Heidenthal (Ed.). *Nursing leadership & management* (pp. 140–156). Clifton Park, NY: Thomson Delmar Learning.

O'Connell, B. (2000). Research shows erosion to advocacy role. *Reflections on Nursing Leadership, 26*(2), 26–28.

Sullivan, E. J., & Decker, P. J. (2001). *Effective leadership and management in nursing* (5th ed.). Upper Saddle River, N.J.: Prentice Hall.

Additional Resources

Anderson, J. E. (2004). Step up to the plate: Participate in political action. *Nursing Matters, 15*(3), 8.

Baldwin, M. A. (2003). Patient advocacy, a concept analysis. *Nursing Standard, 17, 21,* 33–39.

Binstead, R. H. (2001). The politics of caring. In L. E. Cluff, & R. H. Binstock (Eds.). *The lost art of caring: A challenge to health professionals, families, communities, and society.* Baltimore, MD: Johns Hopkins University Press.

Covey, S. (1990). *Principle-centered leadership.* New York: Simon & Schuster.

Davies, C. Political leadership and the politics of nursing. *Journal of Nursing Management, 12*(4), 235–242.

Farfalla, S. (2004). Legislative action & you. Nurse in Washington Internship (NIWI): Legislative internship ignites interest in lobbying for this AHNA member. *Beginnings, 24*(3), 6–7.

Grad, P. A. (2004). Setting future directions at the National Institute of Nursing Research (NINR). *Policy, Politics & Nursing Practice, 5*(2), 95–100.

Marriner-Tomey, A. (2000). *Guide to nursing management and leadership.* St. Louis, MO: Mosby.

McKeon, E., & Artz, M. (2004). Tips for political action. *American Journal of Nursing, 104*(7), 31.

Milstead, J. A. (1999). *Health policy and politics: A nurse's guide.* Gaithersburg, MD: Aspen.

Thompson, L. S. (2003). Use of a university-community collaboration model to frame issues and set an agenda for strengthening a community. *Health Promotion Practice, 4*(4), 385–392.

Trossman, S. (2004). Political action, anyone? *American Journal of Nursing, 104*(7), 73–75.

Web Sites

American Association of Retired Persons
http://www.aarp.org

Nurse in Washington Internship
http://www.nursing-alliance.org/niwi.htm

Consumers for Quality Care
   http://www.consumerwatchdog.org/healthcare

Management of Nursing and Health Care Services: International Council of Nurses
   http://www.icn.ch/psmanagement00.htm

National Institute of Nursing Research
   http://ninr.nih.gov/ninr

Nurse Reinvestment Act
   http://bhpr.hrsa.gov/nursing/reinvestmentact.htm

Policy, Politics & Nursing Practice
   http://www.sagepub.com/journal.aspx?pid=248

CHAPTER 19

NURSING LEADERSHIP AND COLLECTIVE BARGAINING

INTRODUCTION

Labor unions and labor-management relations have a long history in the United States. First formed as craft guilds, unions now represent millions of workers, including many nurses. This chapter outlines the history of collective bargaining and its role in the workplace for nurses now and in the future.

KEY POINTS

1. Definition

    A. **Collective bargaining** is "the practice of employees, as a collective group, bargaining with the management in reference to wages, work practices, and other benefits" (Tazbir, 2003, p. 497)

    B. History of collective bargaining in the United States

        i. began around 1790

        ii. **unions** were originally formed by skilled craftspeople to market and protect their businesses (Sullivan & Decker, 2001)

iii. early federal regulation of collective bargaining (1890–1932)
    a. Sherman Antitrust Act (1890): limited companies' ability to engage in acts designed to lessen or eliminate competition
    b. Clayton Antitrust Act (1914): limited federal courts' abilities to issue **injunctions** (orders issued by a judge at the request of one party that directs another party to refrain from a certain act), thus ending use of Sherman Act against unions
    c. Railway Labor Act (1926): government declared that private employees had the right to join or not join unions, without interference from employers
    d. Norris-LaGuardia Act (1932): denied federal courts the right to issue injunctions in ordinary labor disputes; limited federal jurisdiction in boycotts, pickets, and strikes (Balliet, 1981, cited in Sullivan & Decker, 2001)
iv. federal labor regulations (1935–1974)
    a. National Labor Relations Act (the Wagner Act, 1935): established employees' right to bargain as a group and organize unions; defined unfair employer labor practices (such as discriminating between union and nonunion employees)
    b. Labor Management Relations Act (Taft-Hartley Act, 1947): addressed problems created by Wagner Act by addressing unfair labor union practices; specified unfair labor union practices such as **featherbedding** (requiring that workers be paid for work they did not perform). It empowered the government to obtain an 80-day injunction against any strike that it deemed a peril to national health or safety. This Act also forbade unions from contributing to political campaigns; instead, political action committees must be established without comingling union treasury funds and funds contributed for political action.
    c. Labor Management Reporting and Disclosure Act (Landrum-Griffin Act, 1959): addressed corruption in higher levels of trade union government (Reynolds, et al., 1986, cited in Sullivan and Decker, 2003)
    d. Work Hours Act of 1962: required time-and-a-half pay for work over 8 hours in a day or 40 hours in a week (Columbia 2004)
    e. Occupational Health and Safety Act (1970): created the Occupational Health and Safety Administration (OSHA) and gave OSHA authority to establish safety rules, inspect workplaces for safety violations, and fine companies that violate rules (Columbia, 2004)
    f. Health Care Amendments to Taft-Hartley Act (1974): made employees of private nonprofit hospitals and nursing homes eligible for collective bargaining; outlined a series of dispute-settling procedures to be applied in the health care industry

g. on August 23, 2004, a revision of the Fair Labor Standards Act (FSLA) went into effect. These new regulations may make it easier for RNs to be classified as workers ineligible for overtime pay because it allows exemptions from overtime for workers that lead a team of other employees, which RNs clearly do. Nursing unions are monitoring the workplace to see if RNs are denied overtime pay.

C. Process of unionization

  i. a group of employees decide that they want to be represented by a union

    a. since employees performing different jobs have different needs, bargaining units are usually established; for example, one bargaining unit maybe for registered nurses, another may be for assistive personnel who are not licensed, and another bargaining unit for housekeeping and janitorial staff

    b. bargaining units may or may not be represented by the same union. Some unions restrict membership to a certain category of workers, such as those affiliated with the United American Nurses (an affiliate of the American Nurses Association), that represent only registered nurses through state nurses associations

  ii. select a bargaining agent (union)

    a. called a **representation election**

    b. presided over by the **National Labor Relations Board** (NLRB)

    c. bargaining agent is selected by simple majority of those eligible to join the bargaining unit

    d. nurse managers must remember that during a bargaining agent selection, unfair labor practices apply; managers must ensure that employees' rights to organize are neither interfered with nor are there any repercussions for those who advocate for unionizing

    e. however, there are many reports of "union busting" activities hospitals engage in when nurses attempt to organize, such as threats to employees and firing influential employees who support organizing (Genovese, 2004)

  iii. certification to contract

    a. designation by NLRB that the bargaining unit has the right to enter into a contract with an employer

    b. actual contract must be negotiated, put in writing, and then voted on by union members; the union leaders can make recommendations to members on how they should vote, but all votes are secret

     iv. contract administration
        a. person (one or more people) designated as the union representative (must be a nursing staff member or a union employee) administers the contract
        b. this person's role: to explain contract provisions to the membership and be available to facilitate in the **grievance process**, the formal expressions of misunderstandings or disputes; contract violations; or inadequate labor agreement (Sullivan & Decker, 2001)

D. Grievance process steps

     i. employee talks informally with direct supervisor after an incident has occurred
        a. union representative may be present at the request of the employee who is a union member
        b. written request for action within 10 days
        c. written response required within 5 days
     ii. if response to step 1 does not solve the problem, written appeal is sent to the director of nursing or other designated administrator
        a. employee and union representative are also present at any meetings
        b. administrator must respond within 5 days
     iii. if response to step 2 does not solve the problem, the appeal goes to the director of human resources (same time limits usually apply)
     iv. arbitration: used if previous three steps do not provide resolution
        a. **arbitrator** is a neutral third party
        b. **arbitration** seeks a solution to the problem with benefits to both parties, if possible (Sullivan & Decker, 2001)

E. Collective bargaining: pros and cons

     i. advantages of collective bargaining
        a. standards are guided by contracts
        b. members are able to participate in decision making
        c. union and management must conform to contract
        d. provides workers with more power to assure they are treated fairly and that the process for disciplinary action is open to union oversight
        e. process can question a manager's authority; more people are involved in dispute resolution
        f. union provides collective voice for employees
        g. employees can voice concerns to management without fearing for job security

    ii. disadvantages of collective bargaining
- a. reduced allowance for individual treatment of workers; for example, raises are more likely to be based on objective measurements, such as number of years worked rather than on merit, such as subjective assessments of superior job performance
- b. union members can outvote minority decisions
- c. union members and management must conform to contract
- d. disputes are not handled between employee and management only; thus, there is less room for personal negotiation or judgment and there may be less trust between management and employees when a union is present
- e. union dues must be paid even if a member does not support unionization or union position
- f. individual employees may not agree with collective union voice
- g. unions may not be perceived by all people as appropriate for professionals (Tazbir, 2003)
- h. some people believe that unions inappropriately protect poorly performing workers
- i. some health care professionals are not willing to strike and close down a community's hospital

F. Striking. Because of the critical nature of nursing work, calling a work stoppage, or a **strike**, can be problematic

    i. members of a union are not required to strike, even if a strike is called; however, workers that do not participate and cross a picket line are called "scabs;" there can be a great deal of friction between striking and non-striking workers

    ii. decision to strike must be made by a simple majority of the union members

    iii. many unions make arrangements so that expert nurses are on the picket line at all times; if a critically ill or injured person or woman in labor comes to the hospital, striking nurses will care for these patients until they are stable enough to be transferred to another facility

G. Workplace advocacy

    i. **workplace advocacy**: activities which nurses undertake to address problems in their everyday work setting

    ii. for example, forming a committee to address problems, design alternatives to achieve best patient care, and invent new ways to implement change

    iii. supportive management sees workplace advocacy as positive; management that is strongly authoritative may see these activities as a threat

       iv. in the latter situation, the nurses' recourse may be to engage in collective bargaining (Tazbir, 2003)

H. Nurse manager's role in unionization

       i. nurses have legal authority to participate in collective bargaining in most health care facilities in the United States

       ii. different collective bargaining units may be present in an organization

       iii. nurse managers must be able to manage the differing details and needs of differing bargaining units who have employees on the same nursing unit

       iv. nurse managers should

          a. know the law and ensure that everyone understands both the rights of workers and management

          b. act clearly within the law, even if the organization asks you to defy a contract

          c. try to find out why nurses are asking for collective bargaining if organizing is underway

          d. ensure that employees have access to information that is not pro-union, such as the limits of unions, documented problems with union environments, etc. (Tazbir, 2003)

I. The role of the whistleblower

       i. **whistleblowing** is the "act in which an individual discloses information regarding a violation of a law, rule, regulation, or a substantial and specific danger to public health or safety" (Tazbir, 2003, p. 499)

       ii. health care fraud ranges from filing false claims for reimbursement to performing unnecessary procedures

       iii. as patient advocates, nurses have an ethical and moral duty to protect patients

       iv. whistle-blowing claims (qui tam lawsuits) can be filed on the behalf of the government, the nurse, or the patient

       v. steps for filing whistle-blowing actions include:

          a. file the lawsuit in secret with the court

          b. do not inform the agency or hospital that you have filed the suit

          c. serve a copy of the complaint to the Department of Justice with a written disclosure of all the information discovered

          d. if the government decides to move forward, it will proceed with and pay for the litigation (Tazbir, 2003)

2. Unionization and professionalism

A. Definition of supervisor

     i. according to Title 29 of the U. S. Code, a **supervisor** is "any individual having authority, in the interest of the employer, to hire, transfer, suspend, lay off, recall, promote, discharge, assign, reward, or discipline other employees, or the responsibility to direct them, or to adjust their grievances, or effectively, to recommend such action, if in connection with the foregoing, the exercise of such authority is not of a merely routine or clerical nature, but requires the use of independent judgment" (National Labor Relations Board, 1994, cited in Tazbir, 2004, pp. 506–507)

    ii. because registered nurses supervise others (LPNs, nurses' aides, and assistive personnel) there has been much discussion about whether RNs can legally join a union

   iii. thus, only nurses clearly defined by an organization as employees can unionize

B. Physicians and unions

     i. when physicians are considered employees (such as of an HMO or physicians employed during their residency), they have the ability to join unions

    ii. as with nursing, physicians' discontent about changes in the workplace have led to physicians forming unions

   iii. currently, only about 6 to 10% of physicians are unionized (Charatan, 1999; Sturgeon, 2002)

C. Collective bargaining units for nurses

     i. American Nurses Association (ANA)

       a. ANA represents the nation's entire registered nursing population

       b. mission is to work to improve health care services for all people, foster high nursing standards, and stimulate and promote nurses' professional development

       c. National Labor Relations Board recognizes the United American Nurses (UAN), a full-fledged affiliate of both the ANA and the American Federation of Labor-Congress of Industrial Organizations (AFL-CIO) as a collective bargaining unit in 24 states and the District of Columbia

       d. some believe ANA's dual role and professional organization and collective bargaining unit create conflict; in Massachusetts there are now two state nurses associations—one for collective bargaining—the Massachusetts Nurses Association (MNA), and one for professional development—the Massachusetts Association of Registered Nurses (MARN), the affiliate of ANA

    ii. other labor organizations that represent nurses

       a. American Federation of State, County and Municipal Employees (AFSCME)

b. Service Employees International Union (SEIU)
c. National Nurses Organizing Committee, the newest national union and professional organization for registered nurses and APRNs founded in Spring, 2004 by the California Nurses Association, which is not an affiliate of ANA

D. Major collective bargaining issues for nurses

    i. determining the composition for a collective bargaining unit (since there can be up to 200 different job categories in a hospital)
       a. NLRB established eight eligible health care bargaining units: registered nurses, physicians, all professionals except RNs, technical employees, skilled maintenance employees, clerical employees, guards, and nonprofessional employees
    ii. forming labor-management committees
       a. allow staff nurses and nurse leaders/managers to communicate about issues without entering into a more formal union or grievance procedure
       b. however, these committees have been challenged by unions as violating national labor law
       c. the future impact of the challenges on the workplace is currently unclear (Sullivan & Decker, 2001)
    iii. nurse-patient ratios and what constitutes "safe staffing"

F. Future of collective bargaining

    i. with radical and ongoing changes in the health care environment, collective bargaining holds both concerns and promise for
       a. influencing the practice environment
       b. ensuring economic security for nurses
       c. making patient safety issues and nursing professional development critical elements of labor contracts
    ii. concern is that the collective bargaining process as it exists today may separate rather than unite nurses (Sullivan & Decker, 2001)

REVIEW ACTIVITIES

Questions

1. In the United States, the first unions were formed by groups of craftspeople in which year?

    a. 1790
    b. 1890

    c. 1914

    d. 1935

2. Which of the following legislative acts declared that private employees had the right to join or not join unions without interference from employers?

    a. Clayton Antitrust Act

    b. Railway Labor Act

    c. Norris-LaGuardia Act

    d. Wagner Act

3. This Act allows the government to block a strike for 80 days if it is deemed a peril to national health or safety.

    a. National Labor Relations Act

    b. Taft-Hartley Act

    c. Work Hours Act

    d. Occupational Health and Safety Act

4. The formation of a union and selection of a bargaining agent must be overseen by the:

    a. employer

    b. legislature

    c. National Labor Relations Board

    d. U.S. Department of Labor

5. The formal expressions of misunderstandings, contract violations, or inadequate labor agreements is called:

    a. grievance process

    b. whistleblowing

    c. strike

    d. representation election

6. Activities that nurses undertake to solve problems in their everyday work setting are called:

    a. grievance processes

    b. whistleblowing

    c. workplace advocacy

    d. strikes

7. Which of the following is true about a work stoppage?

    a. it is a necessary part of labor negotiations

    b. if the stoppage is called by the union, all union members must participate

    c. a simple majority vote of union members is required to approve the work stoppage

    d. it will never affect the care of patients

8. Which of the following organizations is a union for registered nurses and an affiliate of the ANA?

    a. UAN
    b. AFSCME
    c. SEIU
    d. NNOC

Critical Thinking Questions

1. Massachusetts and Maine each experienced conflict within their state nurses associations. Nursing unions see management as their adversaries. Yet, state nurses associations that are affiliates of the ANA allow all registered nurses to be members—both management and those represented by the union. Look into the issues that resulted in the formation of two separate organizations in these states. Do you agree with the decision to split? Why or why not?

2. If you were interviewing for a job and the person conducting the interview asked for your opinion about whether nurses should belong to a labor union, how would you respond?

3. There are many unions that represent registered nurses. Compare and contrast the three largest: AFSCME, SEIU, and UAN. Do you believe that one of these unions is better for nurses than another? Why or why not? Support your position with information about the organizations, their history, their mission, and their affiliations.

Discussion Questions

1. Are you a member of a union in your workplace? If so, which one? What benefits does your union provide for you? If given a choice, would you prefer to join a union or not? If you are not a union member, interview a nurse who is a member and ask him or her about union benefits and drawbacks.

2. How does your workplace (or main clinical site) address grievances or disputes? Based on your experience, are these processes effective or ineffective? Why?

3. Should all nurses belong to a union? Why or why not?

Works Cited

Balliet, L. (1981). *Survey of labor relations.* Washington, DC: Bureau of National Affairs.

Charatan, F. (1999). American trade union aims to recruit more doctors. *Western Journal of Medicine, 170*(5), 305–306.

Columbia Electronic Encyclopedia (6th ed.). (2004). U.S. labor law since the early twentieth century. Available online at: http://www.infoplease.com/ce6/bus/A0859157.html Last accessed November 15, 2004.

Genovese, M. (2004) Union-busting industry feeds on lies, distortions. *NYSNA Report, 35*(9), 1, 5.

National Labor Relations Board vs. Health Care & Retirement Corporation of America, U.S., 1124 S.Ct. 1778 (1994).

Reynolds, L. G., Master, S. H., & Moser, C. H. (1986). *Labor economics and labor relations* (9th ed.). Englewood Cliffs, NJ: Prentice-Hall.

Sullivan, E. J., & Decker, P. J. (2001). *Effective leadership and management in nursing* (5th ed.). Upper Saddle River, NJ: Prentice Hall.

Sturgeon, J. (2002). Physicians and unions. *Unique Opportunities* Nov/Dec. Available online at: http://www.uoworks.com/pdfs/feats/UNIONS.pdf. Last accessed November 19, 2004.

Tazbir, J. (2003). Collective bargaining. In P. Kelly-Heidenthal (Ed.). *Nursing leadership & management* (pp. 496–511). Clifton Park, NY: Thomson Delmar Learning.

Additional References

American Nurses Association. *Code of ethics for nurses with interpretive statements.* Washington, DC: American Nurses Publishing; 2001.

Collective bargaining's impact on safe patient care. (2004). *Kentucky Nurse, 52*(2), 7.

Is whistle-blowing really up to me? (2004). *Nursing Standard, 18*(33), 31.

McDonald, S., & Ahern, K. (2002). Physical and emotional effects of whistleblowing. *Journal of Psychosocial Nursing and Mental Health Services, 40*(1), 14.

Polston, M. D. (1999). Whistleblowing: Does the law protect you? *American Journal of Nursing, 99*(1, pt. 1), 26–31.

Salazar, J. (2004). Developing union leaders. *Michigan Nurse, 77*(4), 9.

Slaon, A. J. (2002). Legally speaking. Whistleblowing: Proceed with caution. *RN, 65*(1), 67.

Web Sites

American Federation of State, County and Municipal Employees (AFSCME) http://www.afscme.org

The Burke Group
http://www.djburke.com

Code of Ethics for Nurses
http://www.nursingworld.org/AJN/2001/oct/Issues.htm

National Labor Relations Board
http://www.nlrb.gov

National Nurses Organizing Committee
http://www.nnoc.net

National Whistleblower Center
http://www.whistleblowers.org

PTI Labor Research
http://www.ptilaborresearch.com

Qui Tam Legal Center of Missouri
http://www.qui-tam-law.com

Service Employees International Union
http://www.seiu.org

SEIU Nursing Alliance
http://www.seiu.org/health/nurses

State nurses associations: ANA constituent member list
http://www.nursingworld.org/snaaddr.htm#ma

United American Nurses
http://www.nursingworld.org/uan/about.htm

United Nurses of America (AFSCME)
http://www.afscme.org/una/index.htm

United States Department of Labor Whistleblower Program
http://www.osha.gov/dep/oia/whistleblower/index.html

DELEGATION

assess

clinical experience

delegatee

delegation

evaluate

feedback

intervene

legal issues

noncredentialed assistive personnel

nonunion organization

plan

supervision

unionized organization

INTRODUCTION

One of the key skills of an effective nurse leader is delegating tasks effectively, so that the health care team can provide optimum care for patients. At first glance, it would seem that delegation is a simple task of telling someone to do something. However, delegation requires that the delegator knows laws and regulations, the situation, the institution, and the person to whom the work is assigned. In addition, nurse leaders must supervise, assess, and evaluate delegate performance. This chapter defines delegation and discusses the range of actions that comprise effective delegation.

KEY POINTS

1. **Delegation** is "transferring to a competent individual the authority to perform a selected nursing task in a selected situation. The nurse retains accountability for the delegation." (NCSBN, 1995)

   A. Keys to successful delegation. According to Hansten & Washburn (1998), the activities that make up delegation, like the activities that comprise the nursing process, are cyclical, beginning with gathering and assessing data, through analysis, and so on. The following steps are key to successful delegation:

    i. **assess**, which includes knowing the following components of the practice setting

      a. *environment:* demographic trends, health care delivery trends, changing nature of nursing, changes in nursing population, reimbursement, and regulatory status (Haase-Herrick, 1998)

      b. *organization:* for example, mission, values, quality plans, and delivery systems

      c. *practice:* for example, the state practice act, nursing practice statutes and rules, and institution/organization policies

      d. *self:* including attitudes and beliefs, for example, knowledge of work preferences, or interpersonal barriers that affect delegation

      e. *the delegatee* (person being delegated to): for example, his or her strengths, weaknesses, abilities, preferences, and cultural background; the focus should be primarily on what the person is able to do since it is inappropriate to delegate a task beyond a person's ability

   ii. **plan**

      a. gather information about what needs to be done

      b. prioritize the outcomes that are the most important

  iii. **intervene** (where most delegation "action" takes place)

      a. decide which tasks can be appropriately delegated

      b. communicate effectively (can include instructions, teaching, transfer of skills or other information, and clearly outlining expectations)

      c. resolve conflict (people being delegated to may resist taking on new tasks or learning new skills)

  iv. **evaluate**

      a. oversee the performance of the delegated task

      b. **supervision** is "the provision of guidance or direction, evaluation, and follow-up by the licensed nurse for accomplishment of a nursing task delegated to an unlicensed assistive personnel" (National Council of State Boards of Nursing, 1995, pp. 1–2, cited in Hansten & Washburn, 1998, p. 8)

      c. give feedback to the delegatee about how he or she performs the task, improvements needed, or reinforcing correct performance

      d. problem solving to improve task performance or increase delegatee's understanding

      e. evaluate to ensure the delegatee's competence; in many cases, this step will involve carefully and thoroughly documenting the occurrence and effectiveness of supervision and evaluation

B. The five "rights" of delegation

  i. right task
  ii. right circumstances
  iii. right person
  iv. right direction/communication
  v. right supervision

C. Outcomes of effective delegation

  i. protect patient safety
  ii. achieve desirable patient outcomes
  iii. achieve benefits for the licensed nurse and other personnel
  iv. reduce health care costs by using a mix of personnel appropriately
  v. facilitate access to appropriate level of care
  vi. provide accountability for nursing care
  vii. decrease nurse liability

D. Obstacles to delegation

  i. nonsupportive environment
    a. organizational culture that restricts delegation, for example, due to inflexible hierarchy or management styles
    b. personal qualities, such as poor communication or interpersonal skills
    c. lack of resources
    d. lack of training to teach licensed nursing staff how to delegate appropriately
  ii. insecure delegator
    a. lack of trust between delegator and delegatee
    b. need for approval and affiliation and fear of criticism
    c. fear of liability
  iii. unwilling delegatee
    a. person not willing to take on delegated task due to inexperience, fear of failure, or interpersonal conflict with delegator
    b. delegatee who avoids responsibility (Sullivan & Decker, 2001).

2. Delegation and the health care environment

A. Delegation changes according to changes in the health care environment, such as:

  i. nursing shortage
    a. fewer nurses and more demand for them (since 1980s) leading to use of assistive personnel to help fill the workforce gaps
    b. Bowen Commission (late 1980s) called for innovative use of nursing resources to help offset the shortage (U.S. Department of Health and Human Services, 1998)

      c. Pew Health Professions Commission (1995) recommended that the profession should recover the RN's clinical management role

  ii. health care reform increases need

      a. attempts (for example, the 1996 Kennedy-Kassebaum bill) to provide government-supported health care for certain populations

      b. Medicare: the major purchaser of health care services and products for the growing elderly population

      c. increased number of poor and disabled people receiving health care through Medicaid

      d. cost shifting through premium increases, higher copays, or limiting or controlling access via managed care

  iii. demographic changes and trends (including aging of nurse population)

      a. aging population with the accompanying increase in chronic or debilitating health conditions requiring care

      b. more overall health care expenditures; significant increases in long-term care, home care, supportive care, etc

      c. more people unable to afford health care insurance premiums; people wait longer to seek care and require more care when they do enter the system

      d. increase in use of alternative treatments

      e. consumers more likely to see health care services as "value driven"

      f. increased consumer demand for preventive care and education and increased demand for nurses to provide these services

  iv. increased financial pressures on health care organizations

      a. spiraling care costs mean increased demand for control and accountability

      b. most people now receive care via managed care organizations

      c. significant decrease in length of patient stay in acute care facilities results in much nonacute care moving to other venues (rehabilitation centers, subacute facilities, outpatient care)

  v. changing nature of work

      a. in organizations overall: the loss of job security, flatter organizational structures, frequent mergers and acquisitions, and "outsourcing" of jobs to countries with lower wages and minimal or no benefits

      b. in health care organizations: shortened treatment timeframe from admission to discharge, move to outpatient settings, mergers and acquisitions (fewer community-based hospitals), increased government and payor oversight, closing of hospitals and health care centers for cost reasons

vi. changing nature of health care staffing
  a. for RNs, focus on management and decision making rather than patient care
  b. shift from primarily RN staff to RNs managing a team of assistive personnel (Haase-Herrick, 1998)

B. Delegation and the **unionized organization**

  i. background
    a. American Nurses Association called upon state nurses associations (SNAs) to act as collective bargaining representatives for nurses (1946)
    b. currently, 24 SNAs have full labor relation programs that represent nurses
    c. unions are legally responsible for representing all members fairly; members are responsible for joining and supporting their selected union
    d. nurses delegating must understand the role of the union in ensuring a fair and reasonable working environment
    e. increasing delegatory responsibilities for the RN may make him or her ineligible for representation by a collective bargaining unit if they are classified as working in a supervisory capacity; it may also make RNs ineligible for overtime pay (see chapter 19)

  ii. the impact of the union environment on delegation
    a. employment contracts cover wages, holidays, vacations, benefits, seniority, scheduling, and dispute resolution procedures
    b. contracts cover staffing and patient safety issues, and provide means of maintaining open communication between management and labor
    c. RNs who delegate need to be familiar with contract provisions for the workers to whom tasks are delegated to assure that assignments are consistent with the contract

C. Delegation and the **nonunion organization**

  i. in this environment, ideally
    a. nurses actively participate in committees/task forces, oversee operations, implement needed oversight, and ensure that delegation is performed properly
    b. management provides the tools that staff need to function effectively, including training, and empowers staff to function autonomously
    c. delegation is usually effective due to open communication, ownership and responsibility by staff, and management support to operate most efficiently and cost-effectively (Hansten & Washburn, 1998)

D. Delegation and the individual

    i. effective delegation linked to levels of **clinical experience**

        a. novice: has limited experience with tasks and needs rules to guide actions

        b. advanced beginner: has enough experience to recognize patterns in work; continues to need help setting priorities; relies on rules and protocols

        c. competent: has been practicing 2 to 3 years; can prioritize and cope with various contingencies; requires assistance working through situations not yet experienced

        d. proficient: has enough experience to see the "big picture" rather than series of individual incidents/actions; decision-making is more efficient and accurate; able to prioritize and plan even challenging patient care

        e. expert: no longer relies on rules to understand a situation or to act appropriately; focuses quickly on viable solutions; able to lead a team efficiently, can organize others' work and supervise them effectively (Benner & Benner, 1984, cited in Hansten & Washburn, 1998)

    ii. benefits of delegation

        a. better use of higher-level skills; thus more time for professional nursing tasks

        b. empowerment and most effective use of assistive personnel

        c. less stress from trying to "do it all" and more job satisfaction

        d. greater sense of teamwork and collegial support

    iii. reasons why nurses are reluctant to delegate

        a. averse to taking risks or lack of trust in others; avoiding conflict

        b. difficulty letting go of tasks with personal importance; fear loss of control of tasks and role

        c. requires change in established personal habits and how work is performed

        d. fear that if work/tasks are delegated, the delegator will not be needed

        e. inability to organize or prioritize work that requires others to accomplish

        f. uncertainty about rules and regulations of delegation

        g. lack of leadership and delegation role models (Hansten & Washburn, 1998)

3. Legal issues and delegation

A. Licensure

    i. nurses must know the rules and regulations of their nursing licenses

      ii. proper delegation does not put a nurse's license at risk

    iii. no one works "under" a registered nurse's license except the licensee

B. State boards of nursing

      i. primary goal is protection of the public

     ii. investigate licensed nurses accused of unsafe or illegal practice

    iii. grant or revoke license

    iv. regulate nursing practice

C. Nurse Practice Act

      i. varies by state; basic components include:
        a. defines nursing
        b. sets the licensure process (qualifications, fees, renewals, etc.)
        c. creation of a board of nursing, and defines membership and qualifications
        d. lists powers and duties of the board
        e. grants authority to adopt rules and regulations

     ii. nurse delegator must know practice acts that govern the delegatee

    iii. information is available from the National Council of State Boards of Nursing (www.NCSBN.org) (Hansten & Washburn, 1998)

D. Roles of noncredentialed assistive personnel

      i. **noncredentialed assistive personnel** (NCAP) are:
        a. hired by a health care facility, which defines their scope of practice (within limits of the law)
        b. trained at the facility, by facility personnel, and evaluated at the facility
        c. no external standards apply
        d. no standardized, external evaluation conducted in the form of a standardized credentialing test
        e. may use a variety of titles, including nursing assistant, unit aide, unit tech, nursing tech, etc. (Carroll, 1998)
        f. NCAP term is used instead of "unlicensed assistive personnel" because there are professions in which members are well educated and have a national credential, such as being registered or certified; however, they do not have a state license. The license is not the key differentiation—it is the lack of a credential in the area of practice.

     ii. NCAP role
        a. should be developed in conjunction with the state nursing board to assure that the NCAP functions within appropriate scope of practice
        b. cannot practice nursing without a license to do so

      c. cannot encroach on other professional licenses, such as physical or respiratory therapy or pharmacy

      d. must be directed, supervised and evaluated by an RN, who is ultimately responsible for patient outcome (Carroll, 1998)

4. Delegation in action

  A.   Choosing the right person to delegate

      i. who are the delegatees and what are their roles, for example:

        a. direct care: collecting data, such as vital signs, assisting with activities of daily living, such as walking and personal hygiene, and feeding in selected cases, taking patients to different areas for tests or care, for example; the delegatee collects data and the RN interprets the data

        b. indirect care: activities done on the patient's behalf, such as communicating with team members, gathering supplies, etc

        c. unit-related activities: clerical tasks, ordering supplies, running errands, or attending meetings

        d. personal activities: actions not related to patient care such as meals, breaks, adjusting schedules, or talking with colleagues

        e. documentation: tasks associated with recording patient information, condition, and care provided (Urden & Roode, 1997)

     ii. evaluating delegatee's competence: Is the delegatee competent to perform the task?

        a. requires that standards of competence exist

        b. organization must ensure that competence can be evaluated and measured

        c. competence criteria must meet nursing board standards (Hansten & Washburn, 1998)

    iii. accountability

        a. at the individual level: delegatee performs self-assessment, participates in peer review, and adheres to practice limits, identifies area for improvement

        b. at the organizational level: delegator receives appropriate training, ensures that the standards are upheld, and assesses and evaluates performance

        c. at the regulatory level: board of nursing sets competence standards, communicates them, and uses communication and disciplinary processes to maintain accountability (National Council of State Boards of Nursing, 1997)

        d. if a delegation is made within the organizational expectations of the delegatee and the delegatee provides care below an acceptable standard, it is not the fault of the RN who delegated; for example, if a patient care technician is assigned to take vital signs, knows how to properly measure vital signs, and lies and makes up the numbers, the RN is not liable—the patient care technician is liable for his own behavior and actions

   iv. official and unofficial expectations of job roles
- a. official: as outlined by practice standards and organization's mission and criteria, job descriptions, competency evaluations
- b. unofficial: job tasks such as answering the phone, who is responsible for talking with physicians, are expectations in a workplace but seldom covered in official job descriptions

   v. assessing a delegatee's strengths, weaknesses, motivation, and preferences
- a. usually accomplished through general observation, formal evaluation, such as testing and competency evaluation, and communication with the delegatee
- b. delegatee's perception of activities and the supervisor's evaluation of the activity may not agree
- c. a delegatee who is not performing well needs a clear definition of role, more information, and increased guidance or supervision

   vi. the role of cultural differences and delegation
- a. cultural differences cannot be ignored
- b. communication is key: do not assume that concepts are understood across cultures
- c. learn key features of other cultures (for example, communication issues, space, and time issues) (Hansten & Washburn, 1997; Marthaler, 2003)

B. Role of communication and delegation

   i. effectively communicating to delegatees
- a. may be verbally, in writing, or both
- b. give delegatee a chance to respond

   ii. effectively understanding delegatee responses (verbal and nonverbal)
- a. note discrepancies between verbal and nonverbal messages
- b. note possible effects of delegatee's culture on responses (Marthaler, 2003)
- c. see Chapters 6 and 7 for additional information on effective communication

   iii. effectively assigning tasks
- a. based on delegatee's ability and job description
- b. based on organization's needs and policies

C. Providing **feedback** to delegatees

   i. benefits
- a. RN learns how to lead team
- b. information gathering and learning for both RN and delegatee

      c. reinforce positive performance

      d. open communication allows for better teamwork (Hansten & Washburn, 1997)

   ii. process: **feedback** usually consists of one of four types:

      a. clarifying: restating instructions and making sure there is no confusion

      b. interpretive: observing delegatee's behavior: "I saw you didn't check Mr. Smith's blood pressure. Did you have trouble understanding my instructions?"

      c. judgmental: interpretive, plus drawing conclusions, in the form of a value judgment: "How can we get anything done if you're always taking a break when we're the busiest!"

      d. personal reaction: provides information about personal feelings: "I always feel good when I get to work with you because I know I can count on you." (Hersey & Duldt, 1989)

  iii. upward feedback: allows delegatees to provide open, honest feedback to RN who delegates to them

D. evaluating delegation process

   i. types of evaluation

      a. continuous: checkpoints, timelines, reporting parameters (such as when a certain type of incident occurs)

      b. problem-related: when a problem occurs; uses critical thinking

      c. periodic: on an agreed-upon basis, for example, each shift, after a case is finished, weekly, or monthly

   ii. documenting delegation process

      a. an essential part of effective delegation

      b. may include incident or other reports

      c. should also record process of evaluation and feedback

      d. if a delegatee makes an error, RN must be able to show records that justify why a task was delegated to a particular delegate (Hansten & Washburn, 1998).

REVIEW ACTIVITIES

Questions

1. Transferring the authority to perform a selected nursing task to a competent individual in a selected situation is called:

  a. evaluation

  b. promotion

  c. feedback

  d. delegation

2. The first step to successful delegation is:

   a. plan
   b. intervene
   c. evaluate
   d. assess

3. A registered nurse who is deciding which tasks can be appropriately delegated to an LPN is engaging in which part of the delegation process?

   a. assessing
   b. planning
   c. intervening
   d. evaluating

4. A registered nurse who is prioritizing patient outcomes that are the most important is engaged in which part of the delegation process?

   a. assessing
   b. planning
   c. intervening
   d. evaluating

5. Which of the following is not one of the five "rights" of delegation?

   a. right task
   b. right person
   c. right direction
   d. right experience

6. According to Benner's categories of clinical expertise, a nurse who is able to see the "big picture" rather than a series of individual incidents is at which level?

   a. novice
   b. advanced beginner
   c. proficient
   d. expert

7. Which of the following is true about delegation to a novice?

   a. novices should not be delegated to as they have insufficient experience
   b. novices need rules to guide their actions
   c. novices are able to recognize patterns in their work and can thus handle delegation
   d. novices are able to see the big picture as well as the individual situation

8. Which of the following is a characteristic of noncredentialed assistive personnel?

   a. hired by a state board of nursing
   b. receive training inside the organization that hires them
   c. are governed by external standards set by state nursing boards
   d. are evaluated by state standards

9. Feedback that restates instructions and makes sure there is no confusion is called:
   a. clarifying
   b. interpretive
   c. judgmental
   d. personal feedback

Critical Thinking Questions

1. At Anywhere General Hospital, noncredentialed assistive workers are taught how to measure patients' blood glucose levels by performing a "finger stick" and using a portable measuring device. One of the patients on the unit becomes infected with hepatitis B and an investigation revealed that the assistant never changed gloves between patients. Genetic typing proved that the patient became infected from another patient with diabetes on the unit who had hepatitis B on admission. Is the RN who delegated the task of measuring blood glucose legally liable for the actions of the assistant? Was the delegation appropriate?

2. A key to delegation is to assess the needs of patients and match them with the skills of workers. For example, two men are in the same room and both require someone to feed them. Patient A requires assistance because both of his hands are bandaged following a flash fire when he was working on his car. Patient B requires assistance because he is partially paralyzed following a stroke. Using the steps of appropriate delegation, explain how you would decide whether both, one, or none of the feeding of these two patients can be delegated to a nursing care technician.

3. It is a very busy evening shift on the nursing unit. An RN who is assigned to pass medications is behind and wants to speed up the process. She places each patient's pills in a cup and then, one-at-a-time, hands the cup to an aide in the medication room to take to the patient. Each of the patients for which she does this is able to swallow both the pills and a little water. Is this appropriate delegation? Why or why not?

Discussion Questions

1. How does delegation take place in your organization (or the one in which you have your clinical experience)? Is the delegation process effective or ineffective? Why?

2. Search the Internet for your state's nursing board Web site. What information does it provide?

3. Are you an effective delegator? Based on the information in this chapter, what makes your delegation skills effective or less so? What part of the process needs the most improvement?

4. Think of a supervisor who delegates to you. Is that person an effective delegator? Why or why not? Choose a task and evaluate it based on the process discussed in this chapter. What improvements can you suggest?

Works Cited

Benner, P., & Benner, R. (1984). *From novice to expert: Excellence and power in clinical nursing practice.* Menlo Park, CA: Addison-Wesley Publishing.

Carroll, P. (1998). Buyer beware? Using non-credentialed assistive personnel: Clinical and management perspectives. *Subacute Care Today,* 1(5), 24–28.

Haase-Herrick, K. (1998). Know your world: Why are these changes in my practice happening to me? In R. I. Hansten & M. J. Washburn, *Clinical delegation skills: A handbook for professional practice* (2nd ed.). (pp. 10–47). Gaithersburg, MD: Aspen.

Hansten, R. I., & Washburn, M. J. (1998). *Clinical delegation skills: A handbook for professional practice* (2nd ed.). Gaithersburg, MD: Aspen.

Hersey, P., & Duldt, B. W. (1989). *Situational leadership in nursing.* Norwalk, CT: Appleton & Lange.

Marthaler, M. T. (2003). Delegation of nursing care. In P. Kelly-Heidenthal (Ed.) *Nursing leadership & management* (pp. 266–279). Clifton Park, NY: Thomson Delmar Learning.

McGrath, K. The unionized organization and delegation. In R. I. Hansten & M. J. Washburn (Eds), *Clinical delegation skills: A handbook for professional practice* (2nd ed.). (pp. 83–89). Gaithersburg, MD: Aspen.

National Council of State Boards of Nursing. (1990). *Concept paper on delegation.* Chicago: NCSBN.

National Council of State Boards of Nursing. (December, 1995). Delegation: Concepts and decision-making process. *Issues,* 1–2. Available online at: http://www. ncsbn.org/regulation/uap_delegation_documents_delegation.asp Last accessed November 19, 2004.

National Council of State Boards of Nursing. (1997). *Assuring competence: A regulatory responsibility.* Chicago: NCSBN.

Pew Health Professions Commission (1995). *Reforming health care workforce regulation: Policy considerations for the 21st century.* San Francisco: UCSF Center for the Health Professions.

Sullivan, E. J., & Decker, P. J. (2001). *Effective leadership and management in nursing* (5th ed.). Upper Saddle River, NJ: Prentice Hall.

Urden, L., & Roode, J. (1997). Work sampling. A decision making tool for determining resources and work redesign. *Journal of Nursing Administration, 27*(9), 34–41.

U.S. Department of Health and Human Services. (1998). *Secretary's commission on nursing final report.* Washington, DC: HHS.

Additional Resources

Garvis, M. (2003). Advice of counsel. When it's OK for an RN to delegate. *RN, 66*(12), 70–71.

Hoban, V. (2003). How to enhance your delegation skills. *Nursing Times, 99*(13), 80–81.

Hopkins, D. L. Evaluating the knowledge deficits of registered nurses responsible for supervising nursing assistants: A learning needs assessment tool. *Journal of Nurses Staff Development, 18*(3), 152–156.

Parsons, L. C. (2000). Delegation strategies for registered nurses practicing in turbulent health care arenas. *SCI Nursing, 17*(2), 46–51.

Registered Nurse Utilization of Unlicensed Assistive Personnel. ANA Position Statement. Accessed August 15, 2004 at: http://www.nursingworld.org/readroom/position/uap/uapuse.htm

Registered Nurse Education Relating to the Utilization of Unlicensed Assistive Personnel. ANA Position Statement. Accessed August 15, 2004 at: http://www.nursingworld.org/readroom/position/uap/uaprned.htm

Rhom, L. R. (2002). Delegation of authority. *Undergraduate Nursing, 4*(1), 22–25.

Sheehan, J. P. (2001). Legally speaking. Delegating to UAPs — a practical guide. *RN, 64*(11), 65–66.

Wheeler, J. (2001). How to delegate your way to a better working life. *Nursing Times, 97*(36), 34–35.

Web Sites

Delegation Decision-Making Tree
http://www.ncsbn.org/pdfs/delegationtree.pdf

Delegation Grid: Iowa Nurses Association
http://www.iowanurses.org/delgrid.htm

Delegation in Nursing Online Course: South Dakota State University
http://learn.sdstate.edu/nursing/delegationportalpage.html

National Association of School Nurses: Using Assistive Personnel
http://www.nasn.org/Default.aspx?tabid=201

National Council of State Boards of Nursing
http://www.ncsbn.org

Nurse Delegation: State of Connecticut Department of Mental Retardation
http://www.dmr.state.ct.us/publications/centralofc/hcs_ns97-1.htm

CHAPTER 21

CURRENT AND FUTURE OPPORTUNITIES FOR NURSE LEADERS

INTRODUCTION

In the 21st century, there will continue to be an abundance of opportunities for nurses. Nurses who pursue certification or advanced credentials in addition to their basic nursing education will be positioned to succeed in the rapidly changing health care marketplace. Nurse entrepreneurs, traveling nurses, case managers, and other specialty and advanced practices provide opportunities for nurses to provide and manage care, experience better job and promotion opportunities, and enjoy high levels of job satisfaction.

KEY POINTS

1. Nursing shortages and nursing opportunities

    A.   Data about nurses. As of 2001, nursing **demographics** showed the following:
        i.   average nurse's age: 43
        ii. average age of associate professor of nursing: 52
        iii. enrollment in nursing education programs: decrease of 13%; 1995–1999
        iv. nurses with BS degree: 32%; nurses with MS degree: 10% (National League for Nursing, 2001)

B. **Certification**

    i. "the process by which a nongovernmental agency or association certifies that an individual licensed to practice a profession has met certain predetermined standards specified by that profession for practice" (Jones, 2003, p. 535)

    ii. advantages of certification

        a. allows the nurse to demonstrate knowledge in a specialty area above the basic licensure examination

        b. certifications generally are valid for 5 years and can be renewed

        c. certification may offer more employment and promotion opportunities; some organizations offer a salary differential for certified nurses

    iii. organizations sponsoring certification (partial list): note that the specialty organization itself does not certify; it is an affiliate or subsidiary of the specialty organization

        a. American Association of Nurse Anesthetists

        b. Association of Critical Care Nurses

        c. American Nurses Credentialing Center

        d. National Association of Pediatric Nurses

        e. Wound, Ostomy, and Continence Nurses Society (Jones, 2003)

C. **Traveling nurses**

    i. within the United States

        a. to fill places left open by nursing shortage or other staffing challenges, such as an influx of patients for a finite period of time; for example, the hundreds of thousands of people who spend only the winter months in Florida

        b. usually three-month assignments on the same unit

        c. may travel to various locations throughout the United States, the location is chosen by the nurse and housing is usually provided

        d. traveling nurse company charges the health care organization high rates for the nurse's services

        e. nurses' actual salary maybe similar to other employees or higher, plus benefits including health insurance, vacation pay, referral bonuses and continuing education opportunities

    ii. in other countries

        a. opportunity to travel and experience different cultures

        b. chance to see nursing and medicine practices different from U.S. perspective

        c. positions often advertised in nursing journals and via the Internet

        d. requires person who can adapt to living and working in another culture; may require knowledge of another language (Penny, 1997)

    D.   Nurses as **sales representatives** for medical or pharmaceutical companies

        i. variety of areas in which to work: pharmaceutical, managed care, durable medical equipment, home care

       ii. demand for registered nurses due to their knowledge of pharmacology, technology, patient needs, and health care systems

      iii. perks for working for corporations can include salary, company car, stock options, and performance bonuses

    E.   Nurses as case managers

        i. **case management** is collaborative work with many agencies to produce best outcome for patient (Dickerson, et al., 1999)

       ii. often used for complex cases that require significant amounts of resources and expert coordination of care (for example, trauma from auto accident)

      iii. may involve legal as well as patient care issues

      iv. nurse case manager needs:
          a. expert clinical skills
          b. knowledge of health care system and resources
          c. understanding of health care finances and providers
          d. ability to communicate with a variety of clinical and non-clinical personnel as well as patients and families (Strassner, 1996)

2. Nurse **entrepreneur.** An entrepreneur is a person who organizes and directs a business undertaking, agreeing to experience risk in return for monetary or other rewards

    A.   Benefits and challenges of entrepreneurship

        i. benefits
          a. job satisfaction
          b. flexibility: ability to choose work opportunities and be your own boss

       ii. challenges
          a. working in a competitive market
          b. salary dependent on performance and payment (thus may not be a "payday" every two weeks)
          c. providing own benefits, such as health insurance and disability that an employer usually provides
          d. paying full social security taxes since there is no employer to pay one-half, as is customary
          e. must be able to set goals and accomplish tasks without direct supervision

B. Opportunities

    i. may be inside or outside an organization

    ii. are limited only by the nurse's skills and imagination

    iii. can include technology, adult day care, accreditation, home health, case management, staffing agencies, consulting, continuing education, etc

C. Characteristics of successful nurse entrepreneur

    i. creative and independent

    ii. responsive and accountable (able to manage time, schedule, etc.)

    iii. market savvy and focused on goals

    iv. financial management skills

    v. common sense as well as clinical knowledge

    vi. able to tolerate some risk and manage change positively (Wilson, 1998; Jones, 2003)

    vii. ability to adapt to different working environments and different working relationships

3. Advanced nursing practice

A. What are APRNs?

    i. American Association of Colleges of Nursing task force definition "**Advanced practice nurses** must be master's or doctorally prepared and they must also possess the skills of critical reflective thinking, self-directed learning, and leadership" (O'Flynn, 1996, cited in Jones, 2003, p. 540)

    ii. advanced practice concept began with nurse anesthetists and nurse practitioners; also includes nurse midwife

    iii. advanced practice nurses often focus on prevention, early intervention, and education, and often serve populations left behind by the health care system, including the poor, minorities, uninsured, and chronically ill (Jones, 2003)

B. Clinical nurse specialist

    i. primarily a hospital-based practice

    ii. are registered nurses with advanced nursing degrees, master's degree or doctorate, who are experts in a specialized area of clinical practice

    iii. are usually involved in

        a. staff and patient education

        b. developing care protocols and standards

        c. nursing research

      iv.   they may practice in broader areas, such as critical care or pediatrics, or more narrow areas, such as cardiopulmonary or oncology practices (Jones, 2003)

C.   Certified nurse midwife

      i.   a variety of programs are available; education required varies with program

      ii.   practice in a variety of settings including hospitals, homes, and birthing centers, with nurse-midwife and collaborating physicians agreeing on procedures

      iii.   American Nurses Association also notes that certified nurse midwives are qualified to provide good women's gynecological care and low-risk obstetrical care

D.   Nurse practitioner (NP)

      i.   advance practice nurse with education beyond the bachelor's degree with strong focus on primary care (nurse practitioners who were originally credentialed with less than a Master's degree have been permitted to continue to practice, but all new nurse practitioners must have a Master's degree in order to be licensed)

      ii.   specialized education in diagnosing and treating illnesses and providing health care maintenance

      iii.   depending on state regulations, NP may work independently or may be required to work with a physician

      iv.   state regulations determine whether nurse practitioners can write prescriptions (called "prescriptive authority"); the state also determines which drugs maybe prescribed

      v.   new position: acute care nurse practitioner, who is based in an acute-care setting and combines patient care with prescriptive authority and procedures (such as lumbar puncture) that previously only physicians could do (Jones, 2003)

E.   Certified registered nurse anesthetist

      i.   first recorded nurse anesthetist was in 1877

      ii.   now requires a master's degree

      iii.   takes care of patient's anesthesia needs before, during, and after surgery, either alone or in conjunction with other health care professionals

F.   Wound, ostomy, continence nurse specialist

      i.   care of ostomies as well as skin care, wound and fistula management, care of pressure sores and effects of incontinence

      ii.   may be hospital-based or community-based practice

      iii.   requires bachelor's degree in nursing and enterostomal therapy nursing education program

G.   Flight nursing

    i.   works with critically ill or injured people being transported to hospitals from the scene of an accident or from one hospital to another

    ii.   skills required: endotracheal intubation, EKG interpretation, IV and chest tube insertion, administering medication and sedation, and central line placement

    iii.   usually also requires advanced training such as PALS, ACLS, and NRP (Jones, 2003) and many flight nurse programs require nurses to successfully complete paramedic training

REVIEW ACTIVITIES

Questions

1. The process by which an association affiliate or subsidiary assures that a person has acquired a body of knowledge and has met certain practice standards specified by that organization is called:
    a.   education
    b.   entrepreneurship
    c.   certification
    d.   advanced practice

2. Which of the following is true about certification?
    a.   it allows nurses to demonstrate specific knowledge or clinical experience
    b.   it is usually valid for 10 years
    c.   it is administered by state nursing boards
    d.   it automatically increases a certified nurse's pay

3. This type of nurse coordinates care for complex cases that require significant resources:
    a.   nurse sales representative
    b.   nurse-midwife
    c.   traveling nurse
    d.   nurse case manager

4. A nurse who organizes and directs a business undertaking is called a:
    a.   nurse entrepreneur
    b.   nurse anesthetist
    c.   nurse case manager
    d.   clinical nurse specialist

5. This type of advanced practice nurse usually requires advanced skills such as EKG interpretation, IV and chest tube insertion, and endotracheal intubation.
   a. nurse-midwife
   b. flight nurse
   c. clinical nurse specialist
   d. wound, ostomy, continence nurse specialist

Critical Thinking Questions

1. The Air and Surface Transport Nurses Association made this statement about certification: ". . . certification enables the consumer, the government, third-party payers, and other health-care professionals to identify those who have attained a qualifying level of knowledge" (at http://www.astna. org/Position-papers/FlightNursCert.htm). Do you think certification is important to health care consumers? Does the average patient ever know that nurses can be certified in a specialty? If not, how can they be better informed?

2. Imagine that you want to set up a business as a nurse consultant in wound care. In order to market yourself and create a financially viable business, answer the following questions:
   a. Why is a nurse qualified to be a wound care consultant?
   b. What services could you offer?
   c. Which people, companies, or organizations might be interested in your services?
   d. Why would a client want to hire a nurse instead of a physician?
   e. How can a nurse consultant save the client money?
   f. Is it important for the nurse consultant to be certified? Why?
   g. How can the nurse establish his or her expert credentials?
   h. How can a new nurse consultant find other nurse entrepreneurs with whom he can build a network?

Discussion Questions

1. What type of advanced nursing practice most interests you? What additional skills and education would you need to pursue this practice?

2. Name your entrepreneurial qualities. What type of entrepreneurial nursing role would you be interested in pursuing? Why?

Works Cited

Dickerson, P. S., Peters, D., Walkowiak, J. A., & Brewer, C. (1999). Active learning strategies to teach case management. *Nurse Educator, 24*(5), 52–57.

Jones, S. (2003). Emerging opportunities. In P. Kelly-Heidenthal (Ed.). *Nursing leadership & management* (pp. 532–550). Clifton Park, NY: Thomson Delmar Learning.

National League for Nursing. (2001). Press release. Accessed August 15, 2004 from www.nln.org/.

O'Flynn, A. (1996). The preparation of advanced practice nurses. *Nursing Clinics of North America, 31*, 429–448.

Penny, J. T. (1997). What a travel nurse company seeks in you. *Nursing 1997, 27*(6), 69.

Strassner, L. F. (1996). The ABCs of case management: A review of the basics. *Nursing Case Management, 1*(1), 22–30.

Wilson, C. K. (1998). Mentoring the entrepreneur. *Nursing Administration Quarterly, 22*(2), 1–12.

Additional Resources

American Nurses Association (January, 2004). Career Guide, 2004. *American Journal of Nursing, 16*.

Cramer, M. E., Chen, L. W., Mueller, K. J., Shambaugh-Miller, M., & Agrawal, S. (2004). Predictive Model to Determine Need for Nursing Workforce. *Policy, Politics & Nursing Practice, 5*(3). 174–192.

Whitehead, D. (2003). The health-promoting nurse as a health policy career expert and entrepreneur. *Nurse Education Today, 23*(8), 585–592.

Wilson, A. (2003). The influences on and experiences of becoming nurse entrepreneurs: A Delphi study. *International Journal of Nursing Practice, 9*(4), 236–245.

Your guide to certification: Here's what you need to know to pursue additional credentials. (January, 2004). *American Journal of Nursing*, 58–70.

Web Sites

American Association of Nurse Anesthetists
    http://www.aana.com

Association of Critical Care Nurses
    http://www.aacn.org

American Nurses Credentialing Center
    http://www.ana.org/ancc

Healthcare Traveler
  http://www.healthcaretraveler.com/healthcaretraveler/

Society of Psychiatric Advanced Nurse Practitioners
  http://www.njsna.org/society_of_psychiatric_advanced_.htm

Travel Nurses
  http://www.travelnursing.com

Wound, Ostomy, and Continence Nurses Society
  http://www.wocn.org

Nurse Entrepreneur Web Sites: Ed4Nurses
  http://www.ed4nurses.com

Great Nurses
  http://www.greatnurses.com/

National Nurses in Business Association
  http://www.nnba.net/

Neuroscience Nursing Consultants
  http://www.neuronurse.com/index.html

Nurse's Notebook, LLC
  http://www.nursesnotebook.com

Nursing NowNotes
  http://www.nursingnownotes.com/index.asp

Part V

Legal and Ethical Aspects of Nursing Leadership

CHAPTER

22 LEGAL ASPECTS OF NURSING LEADERSHIP

INTRODUCTION

Laws govern our conduct and protect us from harm. But what if the nurse is the one accused of "doing harm"? This chapter discusses the legal aspects of providing nursing care, including areas of liability and ways for nurses to decrease their risks of lawsuits.

KEY POINTS

1. Definitions and categories

    A.   **Laws** are "rules of conduct, established and enforced by authority, which prohibit extremes in behavior so that one can live without fear for oneself or one's property" (Sullivan & Decker, 2001, p. 71)

    i. **public law** consists of constitutional law, criminal law, and administrative law

    ii. **civil law** governs how people relate to each other in everyday matters, and consists of contract law and tort law

    iii. nurses can be affected by:

        a. criminal law: if they commit a criminal act or are victims of a crime

        b. administrative law: such as federal regulations that prevent discrimination due to age or disability

        c. civil law: specifically tort law

B. Tort law

    i. a **tort** is a "private or civil wrong or injury, including action for bad faith breach of contract, for which the court will provide a remedy in the form of an action for damages" (*Black's Law Dictionary*, 1996, cited in Martin & Cain, 2003)

    ii. a tort can be any of the following:

        a. denial of person's legal rights

        b. failure to comply with public duty

        c. failure to perform private duty that harms another person

    iii. tort can be unintentional (such as malpractice or neglect) or intentional (such as assault and battery) (Fiesta 1999)

    iv. tort charges that a nurse can face include assault and battery, false imprisonment, invasion of privacy, defamation, and fraud (Martin & Cain, 2003)

    v. tort reform is an ongoing political and legal issue that is hotly debated. See "Tort Reform" Web sites, at the end of this chapter.

C. Regulation of nursing practice

    i. the law that defines and regulates nursing practice is called the **Nurse Practice Act**

    ii. each state establishes its own rules and regulations

    iii. the Nurse Practice Act establishes the scope of practice for licensed practical nurses and registered nurses and differentiates the practice of nursing from the practice of medicine

D. Definitions of negligence and malpractice

    i. **negligence** is "the failure of an individual not to perform an act (omission) or to perform an act (commission) that a reasonable, prudent person would or would not perform in a similar set of circumstances" (Sullivan & Decker, 2001, p. 75)

    ii. **malpractice** is professional negligence and refers to "any misconduct or lack of skill in carrying out professional responsibilities" (Sullivan & Decker, 2001, p. 75)

    iii. for malpractice to exist, the following elements must be present:

a. a duty exists: this is automatic when a patient is in a health care facility or the patient of an organization such as a home care company
b. a breach of duty occurs: the nurse did something that shouldn't have been done, or didn't do something that should have been done
c. causation: the nurse's action directly led to a patient injury
d. injury: harm that comes to the patient
e. damages: compensate patient for injury

2. Legal issues specific to nursing

A. **Patient care issues**

   i. medication and IV errors
      a. wrong medication or incorrect dosage
      b. wrongly administered
      c. wrong patient
      d. administering a medication to which a patient has a known allergy
   ii. injuries
      a. caused by equipment used: Safe Medical Devices Act (1990) requires that any equipment malfunction that causes serious injury, illness or death must be reported to the FDA and the manufacturer within 10 days
      b. caused by restraints placed on a patient: Omnibus Budget Reconciliation Act (OBRA) of 1997 requires that restraints be used only as a last resort, and used only under a physician's order
      c. falls
   iii. responsibility
      a. patient is prematurely discharged: assessing patient's condition at discharge is nurse's responsibility
      b. patient refusing care: nurses must act to protect patient (informed consent, informing about results of nontreatment) and protect self (charting consent attempts and patient's refusal)
      c. nurse fails to follow up with physician or other health care providers when there is a change in patient's condition
   iv. errors due to language barriers
      a. physicians and staff from other countries
      b. patients whose primary language is not English
      c. both JCAHO and American Hospital Association require hospitals to meet patient's communication needs
      d. possible solutions include instructions in other languages; having staff serve as interpreters when appropriate and developing a policy to enhance communication

    v. home care
- a. essential to know the chain of command for notifying supervisors and physicians of change in patient status
- b. nurse must be aware of how patient equipment (such as home ventilator or infusion device) works, and how to ensure that the equipment functions properly
- c. appropriate delegation to assistive staff: for example, does a home aide know enough to respond appropriately to a patient who develops shortness of breath? (Sullivan & Mattera, 1997)

B. Surrounding **documentation** and charting

    i. rules for appropriate documentation and charting (electronic or written) include
- a. chart all interventions
- b. spell out instructions and discharge planning
- c. be sure to identify an assessment of patient understanding, particularly of discharge instructions, whether from inpatient care or day surgery or the ED

    ii. charting "do's"
- a. limit use of abbreviations to those approved by the organization
- b. include time, date, and signature on each entry
- c. follow hospital policy regarding corrections/deletions/amendments

    iii. charting "don'ts"
- a. don't use the chart to accuse or blame others
- b. record observations such as: "entered room and found patient on floor" rather than conclusions: "patient fell out of bed"
- c. describe a patient's behavior: "patient raised voice and made a fist" rather than labeling as "uncooperative" or "combative"
- d. don't be afraid to amend the chart, using approved procedures, to clarify or provide more information

    iv. common charting omissions that should be included:
- a. abnormal vital signs and nursing actions taken
- b. in cardiac arrest: provide details about events leading up to the event and how patient and family were taken care of after the event; this in addition to the code record
- c. when a patient is transferred: be sure to note when the report was given and to whom; for transfer to another facility (except for transport to the ED for urgent or emergent care) note the names of the nurse and the physician accepting the transfer
- d. patient teaching: including what information was provided and assessment of patient understanding
- e. patient's refusal of treatment: use forms according to policy and document in detail the events leading to the patient refusal,

the information provided that explains the consequences of refusal, and that there were no repercussions as a result of the patient refusal

    f. any instructions relayed by telephone or e-mail—were the instructions a result of a patient inquiry, or was the contact initiated by the nurse?

  v. documenting incidents and incident reports

    a. generally an internal procedure but can be used in court in limited circumstances

    b. accurately record all details (time, date, patient's name, family notification, physician notification)

    c. provide objective description of incident and any actions taken in response

    d. never provide information about how the incident could have been avoided; if this is used in court, and a document lists this information, the opposing attorney will then be able to ask why the nurse did not take those actions since he or she knew how to prevent the incident

    e. document patient assessment and monitoring after the incident

    f. if the nurse is not sure whether information should be included, check with the nurse manager, supervisor, or risk manager before making a permanent record

  vi. the dangers of **charting by exception,** an approach in which only "out of the ordinary" findings are charted

    a. some organizations adopted this method to save time

    b. does not provide evidence of appropriate nursing care provided

    c. thorough charting means safer patient care and sounder evidence in case of litigation (Sullivan & Mattera, 1997)

C. Legal risks and issues of **telephone triage**

  i. in the best interest of the patient, nurses should avoid giving advice over the phone (Emergency Nurses Association, 1996) unless in a position as an advice nurse

  ii. use protocols such as symptom-based protocols and standing orders for consistency and legal protection

  iii. attempt to ensure the patient's understanding and compliance once instructions are given

  iv. document all aspects of the conversation, including the question asked by the patient, signs, symptoms and advice given (Sullivan & Mattera, 1997)

D. Ground rules for effective nurse-physician-patient communication

  i. nurse must communicate accurately both verbally and in writing

  ii. in many legal cases, lack of communication is cited as a major factor in litigation

      iii. nurse should immediately document all incidents and changes in patients' conditions

      iv. charting should be factual, legible, have no erasures, and be accurate and complete (Martin & Cain, 2003)

E. **Patient Self-Determination Act** (PDSA) (effective December 1991).

    i. goal of PSDA

      a. to make it easier for patients to express their preferences about medical treatment (especially end-of-life care)

      b. to make it easier for health care providers to honor those preferences

      c. primary methods are living wills and durable powers of attorney for health care, also known as health care proxies

      d. nurses are required to ask patients if they have advance directives when they enter the health care system or are admitted to a health care facility if the facility receives federal funds

    ii. how nurses can work with patients and families effectively

      a. find out about the advanced directive statutes in practice area

      b. speak to the risk manager, nursing administrator, patient advocate or chaplain about providing forms for patients

      c. help develop a policy that allows patients to discuss directives in the most appropriate place

      d. establish ways in which the documents can become part of the medical record and assure that they will not be overlooked if there is a sudden or unexpected change in patient's condition

      e. encourage organization to be an educator on this issue and inform the community (Sullivan & Mattera, 1997)

3. Nurses' rights and responsibilities

A. Injuries caused by a patient

    i. nurse has the right to press charges if the patient threatens or intentionally injures the nurse (patient's competency maybe at issue during an investigation)

    ii. nurses are entitled to worker's compensation when injured by a patient (intentionally or not)

B. Matching assignments and skills

    i. nurses can refuse an assignment that is beyond their scope of practice or skill level

      a. decision should be in the best interest of the patient

      b. backup documents are the employee manual and the state's Nurse Practice Act

    c. nursing unions have forms and special procedures to protect nurse members from unsafe assignments

    d. nurse must be aware that refusing an assignment can constitute patient abandonment and may have serious consequences including disciplinary action and reports to the state board of nursing

  ii. nurses should feel free to question a supervisor who assigns a task for which the nurse is not prepared or qualified

    a. communicate clearly why the task poses a risk to patients

    b. explore alternatives such as cross-training in preparation for future assignments or performing other tasks

C. Refusing an assignment

  i. nurses have the right to refuse any assignment they ethically oppose (American Nurses Association, 1995; JCAHO, 1997)

  ii. right to refusal can be based on religious beliefs or on a "conscience" basis, which includes ethical decisions

  iii. the law is less clear about nurse's rights when the refusal is because the nurse believes that the nurse to patient ratio is unsafe; that is, too many patients for one nurse to care for properly

D. When nurses disagree with physicians

  i. nurse's job is to speak up for the patient

  ii. all state laws uphold the right and responsibility of the nurse to question any practice that is inappropriate, incompetent, unethical, or illegal

  iii. nurses should use chain of command when appropriate, and document contact with physicians (Sullivan & Mattera, 1997)

E. Sexual harassment and job discrimination

  i. **sexual harassment** is defined as unwanted sexual advances, requests for sexual favors, and other verbal or physical conduct of a sexual nature

    a. quid pro quo: when a supervisor makes submission to sexual demands a requirement for continued employment or basis for employment decisions, such as promotions, transfers, or scheduling requests

    b. hostile environment: when someone's sexual conduct is pervasive or severe enough to intimidate or offend an employee, or interfere with his or her ability to perform the job; for example, offensive pictures or poster in work area or break room; sexualized atmosphere due to employees telling obscene jokes

  ii. actions to take when harassed

    a. confront the harasser and state clearly and explicitly that the attention is unwanted

        b. report the behavior to a supervisor (or higher if the harasser is the supervisor)

        c. document the harassment

        d. seek support (American Nurses Association, 1993)

        e. if the harasser is a patient, tell the patient that the conduct is inappropriate, then notify other nurses and supervisor

        f. if the harasser is a physician, notify the nursing chain of command and if no resolution, make a report to the medical chief of staff

    iii. manager's role in protecting staff from harassment

        a. employers are liable for harassment by supervisory personnel

        b. employers should have written policies on sexual harassment

        c. any allegations must be handled promptly and discreetly (EEOC, 1980)

  F. Personal disability and family leave

    i. Americans with Disabilities Act (ADA) prevents discrimination on the job based on disability (physical or mental impairment that substantially limits at least one major life activity) (ADA, 1990)

    ii. nurses who believe that they have been discriminated against should seek immediate resolution from the employer; if no resolution, contact the EEOC, the employee collective bargaining unit, or an employment lawyer

    iii. family and Medical Leave Act of 1993 protects the nurse's job when time is taken off for childbirth, adoption, foster care placement, to care for a family member with a serious health condition, or due to the nurse's own health condition

    iv. length of leave time allowed varies according to how "work week" is defined by job, hours usually worked, etc

    v. people who work for small companies (50 or fewer employees) may not be covered

4. Protecting **nursing license**

  A. Actions to avoid

    i. negligence

    ii. incompetence

    iii. abusive behavior

    iv. drug and alcohol abuse/impairment

    v. physical or mental impairment

    vi. fraud

  B. Understanding **disciplinary procedures**

    i. complaint made to the state board of nursing about nurse's action (or inaction) triggers investigation

        a. most boards ask nurse to provide a written response to the complaint

        b. nurse should consult an attorney and phrase an objective response; since the nurse's license and livelihood are at risk, nurses should never enter this process without their own legal representation

        c. avoid talking to anyone about the case without the attorney's approval

  ii. investigation findings are reviewed by the state nursing board

        a. if investigation finds that the complaint has merit, it may schedule a hearing, or allow the nurse to sign a consent agreement to avoid time and expense of a trial

        b. if the nurse decides to fight the complaint with a defense before the board, the nurse works with the attorney to prepare a defense

  iii. decisions by state nursing board

        a. censure: board states disapproval of nurse's actions and records this in the minutes

        b. letter of reprimand: a more severe expression of disapproval of nurse's actions

        c. probation: nurse's professional activities are closely monitored for a period of time

        d. license suspension: nurse prohibited from practicing for a period of time

        e. license revocation: the most severe penalty; prohibits the nurse from ever practicing again

  iv. if the nurse disagrees with the board's decision, the nurse can appeal in trial court (Sullivan & Mattera, 1997)

  v. boards of nursing can take action against a nurse's license for crimes committed outside of nursing practice, such as driving while intoxicated, fraud, resisting arrest, petty larceny, and sexual abuse (for an example of disciplinary actions taken against nurses, visit http://www.op.nysed.gov/jul04.htm#nurse)

C. Other legal situations

  i. giving a deposition

        a. notify the lawyer and the insurance carrier but avoid discussing the case with others

        b. keep answers brief and to the point; provide only the amount of information required to answer the question

        c. be aware of body language and be consistent with verbal message

  ii. acting as an expert witness

        a. expert witness is the only person whose opinion counts as evidence in a legal proceeding

    b. expert witnesses are required to explain why a professional's conduct fell below acceptable standards of practice because a lay jury would not otherwise be able to determine if conduct was appropriate or inappropriate

    c. only nurses can testify as to the appropriate practice of a nurse

    d. each side in a case will have an expert that supports their interpretation of the facts; the judge or jury determines which expert is more believable

    e. nurses should decide if their background and experience qualifies them to offer an informed opinion about another nurse's practice; ultimately, they will be qualified by the court

    f. being an expert witness is part of being a nurse leader—to help defend nurses from unfair allegations and to help expose nurses whose practice is harmful to patients

5. Other legal risks/issues for nurses

  A. **Managed care.** Current areas for concern include:

    i. premature discharge

      a. discharge decisions increasingly being made at administrative level rather than at the bedside

      b. nurse's responsibility to assess the patient's status at discharge

      c. nurses should also know key decision makers (usually utilization review coordinator or case manager) so that the nurse can report concerns directly to them

      d. nurses should also report concerns to physicians but should be aware that physicians are under pressure from managed care networks to cut patient length of stay

      e. patients are informed that if they remain in the hospital, they will be personally responsible for all charges; so many patients will leave whether it is appropriate or not because they cannot afford to pay

    ii. downsizing

      a. fewer RN staff

      b. increased number of assistive personnel

      c. nurse managers need to make sure that delegation is appropriate (see Chapter 20 on delegation)

    iii. emergency care

      a. emergency departments are required by law to treat people who come to the ED and to stabilize their conditions before any transfer is contemplated

      b. managed care companies may refuse to pay for visits, care and/or tests that they consider nonemergency

      c. some legislation has been enacted to require that coverage decisions be made on the patient's symptoms on arrival for care, not the final diagnosis (for example, chest pain that turns out to be a muscle pull may not qualify for reimbursement if only the diagnosis is considered, but chest pain could also be from a myocardial infarction, and patients should be encouraged to seek care for potentially life-threatening symptoms)

    d. nurses should know their organization's policies and procedures for ED care

B.   HIV/AIDS

    i. confidentiality and HIV status; all states report to the Centers for Disease Control and Prevention, but states differ in terms of notification of other parties such as sexual partners

    ii. nurses should know their state's and organization's policy on confidentiality and conform to it

    iii. health care providers have been sued successfully for damages for breaching the confidentiality of patients who are HIV positive (for a report on a breach by a nurse's aide, see Smith & Berlin, 2001)

C.   **Do not resuscitate (DNR) orders**

    i. standard of care requires that nurses must attempt to resuscitate patients who do not have a DNR order

    ii. nurses may find themselves in conflict if, as patient care advocates, they determine that resuscitation is inappropriate

    iii. a proactive approach such as dealing with DNR issues before a crisis occurs remains the best option for nurses; for example, through advance directives

    iv. nurses should be familiar with their organization's policies and procedures, as well as their state nursing board's position on these issues (Sullivan & Mattera, 1997)

D.   **Telemedicine**

    i. also called telehealth, teleconsults, electronic medicine, telemetry, telephone triage

    ii. uses communications technology to transmit health information from one location to another

    iii. legal issues include:

        a. providing care across state lines, since most nurses are licensed in their state of residency (see multistate practices, page 282)

        b. ensuring that patients are making informed consent (usually through both spoken and written channels)

        c. confidentiality: maintaining existing confidentiality measures as well as ensuring security of electronic transmissions (Sullivan & Mattera, 1997; Telemedicine Research Center, 1997)

E. **Multistate practices/compacts**

    i. mutual state recognition model of nurse licensure

    ii. allows nurse to have one license (in his or her state of residence) and practice in other states (both physical and electronic)

    iii. subject to each state's Nurse Practice Act

    iv. each participating state has a Nurse Licensure Compact Administrator to facilitate information exchange (Nurse Licensure Compact, n.d.).

6. Current legal protections for nurses

A. **Good Samaritan laws**

    i. enacted to protect the health care professional from legal liability to encourage such professionals to offer help in emergency or accident situations

    ii. Good Samaritan laws are enacted when

        a. care is rendered in an emergency

        b. health care worker is rendering care without pay

        c. care provided did not recklessly or intentionally harm the injured person (Martin & Cain, 2003)

B. Skillful communication includes:

    i. notifying physician of anything significant that the patient or family has notified the nurse about or that the nurse has observed

    ii. charting all actions, including:

        a. clear and thorough information about observation and notification

        b. date and time notation by the entry

        c. document all attempts to pass on information

        d. avoid phrases such as "communicated with Dr. Jones." Be specific: "Patient's blood pressure increased to 180/110. Call placed to Dr. Jones at 1800 hrs. Left message with answering service, advising him that there was a change in Mr. Levy's condition, requesting a call back. . ." (Sullivan & Mattera, 1997)

C. Excellent relationships with patients and families

    i. many cases that go to court are prompted by a patient's or family's sense that they did not receive proper information or attention from nurses and/or physicians

    ii. nurses should always work to communicate clearly to patients and their families, while making sure that the patient's confidentiality is maintained

      iii. all attempts to contact a patient or family member, as well as conversation with them, their concerns, and nurse's responses should be clearly and carefully documented (Sullivan & Mattera, 1997)

D. **Risk management**

      i. designed to identify and correct system problems that contribute to errors in patient care or employee injury

      ii. emphasis is on quality improvement and protecting the organization from the financial liability of litigation

      iii. most organizations have tracking forms that document incidents, called incident reports

      iv. after an incident, the risk management department will attempt to identify the cause of the incident and implement appropriate action (for example, change in processes, education, employee discipline, etc.) to prevent a recurrence

      v. these remedies are clearly documented as well and kept on file in case of later legal action (Martin & Cain, 2003)

E. Malpractice insurance

      i. nurses should carry their own malpractice insurance, which pays for an attorney to exclusively represent the nurse in a malpractice lawsuit or action in front of the state board of nursing

      ii. not enough to rely on institution's insurance

      iii. the institution may deny the nurse defense if the nurse was not acting according to the organization policy or was acting outside the scope of practice, or if the institution's interests are at odds with the nurse's interests

F. The following suggestions apply to consulting and collaborating with an attorney:

      i. retain a specialist if you have a choice of counsel

      ii. be attentive and involved: read documents provided by the attorney, travel to court proceedings to observe the attorney

      iii. notify insurance carrier as soon as a potential liability issue arises

      iv. ask for specific information (preferably in writing) about how fees will be computed and billed; be sure to ask about expense policies and retainers

      v. attorney should provide copies of all correspondences, legal briefs, and other relevant documents

      vi. stay in touch: the attorney should answer questions promptly and send updates about the case's progress

      vii. if needed, make corrections on draft documents; and deposition transcripts initial any changes (LaDuke, 2000)

REVIEW ACTIVITIES

Questions

1. A rule of conduct that prohibits extremes in behavior so that people can live their lives without fear for self or property is called:
   a. the Nurse Practice Act
   b. a law
   c. advance directives
   d. a DNR order

2. Constitutional, criminal, and administrative law all fall in the category of:
   a. civil law
   b. public law
   c. state law
   d. contract law

3. Tort law is a part of:
   a. civil law
   b. administrative law
   c. criminal law
   d. constitutional law

4. This refers to any misconduct or lack of skill in carrying out professional responsibilities.
   a. negligence
   b. malpractice
   c. standard of practice
   d. assault and battery

5. Which of the following is true about appropriate charting?
   a. record assessment findings and related interventions
   b. erase mistakes to assure a correct record
   c. record interpretations and conclusions about facts
   d. use abbreviations as much as possible

6. This act's goal is to make it easier for people to express their preferences about medical treatment, especially terminal care.
   a. Americans with Disabilities Act
   b. Family Leave Act
   c. Patient Self-Determination Act
   d. Nurse Practice Act

7. Which of the following statements is correct about a nurse's rights and responsibilities?

a. nurses should avoid questioning a supervisor or doctor who assigns a task
b. care decisions should be made in the best interest of the patient
c. nurses can press charges against every patient who threatens to harm them
d. a nurse cannot file for workers' compensation if injured by a psychotic patient

8. A supervisor who tells a nurse that she must meet his sexual demands in order to keep her job is guilty of:

a. creating a hostile environment
b. quid pro quo sexual harassment
c. malpractice
d. breach of duty

9. Which of the following is a legal risk for nurses working in a managed care environment?

a. premature discharge
b. patient teaching
c. emergency care
d. multistate compacts

10. If a nurse renders assistance in an emergency, the injured person cannot sue the nurse due to which of the following?

a. telemedicine regulations
b. multistate compacts
c. Good Samaritan laws
d. Nurse Practice Act

Critical Thinking Questions

1. Disciplinary actions taken against nurses by most state boards of nursing are published, either in newsletters or online or both. Do you agree that this information should be made public? Why or why not? What is the practice in your state?

2. Most states have a mechanism in place whereby nurses with substance abuse problems can admit they have a problem and register with the state board of nursing. By entering the state's program, the nurse's confidentiality is maintained and the license is suspended during treatment. What is your state's program called? How can a nurse enter the program? What are the requirements to resume the practice of nursing after treatment?

3. A nursing unit has two patients with the last name of Smith. James Smith has an order for 2 acetaminophen tablets to treat a fever. The nurse gives

John Smith the acetaminophen instead. John Smith suffers no untoward effects from receiving the acetaminophen erroneously. Do these facts support bringing a malpractice action against the nurse? Why or why not?

Discussion Questions

1. What are your institution's policies and procedures for charting? Correcting errors? Documenting incidents? Based on what you have learned, are these procedures adequate to protect nurses in your organization? If not, what needs to be improved?

2. Interview a nurse in your area who uses telemedicine or does telephone triage. What policies and procedures are in place for his or her protection?

3. Is your state part of a Boards web site multistate agreement? Go to the National Council of State Nursing Boards to find out. Would you prefer to work in a state that is part of such an agreement? Why or why not?

4. What are the nurses' disciplinary procedures in your state? (see the Web site for your state nursing association/board).

Works Cited

American Nurses Association. (1993). *Sexual harassment: It's against the law* (Item WP-3). Washington, DC: Author.

American Nurses Association. (1995). *Code for nurses with interpretive statements*. Kansas City, MO: Author.

Americans with Disabilities Act of 1990. Pub. L. 101–336, 104 Stat. 327.

Emergency Nurses Association. (1996). *Emergency Nurses Association position: Telephone advice*. Park Ridge, IL: Author.

Equal Employment Opportunity Commission. (1980). *Guidelines on discrimination because of sex*. 45 FR 74677, Nov. 10, 1980.

Fiesta, J. (1999). Do no harm: When caregivers violate our golden rule, part 1. *Nursing Management, 30*(8), 10–11.

Joint Commission on Accreditation of Healthcare Organizations. (1997). 1996 *Accreditation manual for hospitals*, Vol. 1, Standards. Oakbrook Terrace, IL: Author.

LaDuke, S. (2000). What should you expect from your attorney? *Nursing Management, 31*(1), 10.

Martin, J. W., & Cain, K. (2003). Legal aspects of patient care. In P. Kelly-Heidenthal (Ed.). *Nursing leadership & management* (pp. 446–463). Clifton Park, NY: Thomson Delmar Learning.

Nurse Licensure Compact. (n.d.) Accessed August 16, 2004 at: http://www.ncsbn.org/nlc/index.asp

Smith, J. J., & Berlin, L. (2001). The HIV-positive patient and confidentiality. *American Journal of Roentgenology, 176*,599–602. Available at: http://www.ajronline.org/cgi/content/full/176/3/599

Sullivan, E. J., & Decker, P. J. (2001). *Effective leadership and management in nursing* (5th ed.). Upper Saddle River, NJ: Prentice Hall.

Sullivan, G. H., & Mattera, M. D. (Eds.) (1997). *Legally speaking: How to protect your patients and your license.* Montvale, NJ: Medical Economics.

Telemedicine Research Center. (1997). *What is telemedicine?* Portland, OR.

Additional Resources

Ashley, R. C. (2004). The Third Element of Negligence. *Critical Care Nurse, 24*(3), 65–67.

Benko, L. B. (June 28, 2004). New call for patients' bill of rights. *Modern Healthcare, 34*(26), 12.

Berry M. (2004). Legally speaking. Saying the right thing when things go wrong. *RN, 67*(4), 59, 61, 63.

Brooke P. S. (2004). Legal questions. Emergency intervention: Stretching the Good Samaritan law. *Nursing, 34*(7), 22.

Brooke, P. S. (2004). What's wrong with this pitcher? *Nursing, 34*(8), 28.

Brooke, P. S. (2003). How good a Samaritan should you be? *Nursing, 33*(6), 46–47.

Edmunds, M. W., & Yeo, T. P. (2004). What to expect from medical liability tort reform. *Nurse Practitioner, 29*(5), 7.

Klutz, D. L. (2004). Tort reform: An issue for nurse practitioners. *Journal of the American Academy of Nurse Practitioners, 16*(2), 70–75.

Mackay, T. (2004). Advice of counsel. The wrong way to amend the medical record. *RN, 67*(6), 57, 64–65.

Mott, J. (2003). Older and unemployed. *Nursing, 33*(11, part 1), 8.

Valente, S. M., & Bullough, V. (2004). Sexual harassment of nurses in the workplace. *Journal of Nursing Care Quality, 19*(3), 234–242.

Web Sites

AIDSLaw of Louisiana: Confidentiality vs. Duty to Warn
    http://www.aidslaw.org/confident.htm

American Nurses Association Code of Ethics
    http://www.ana.org/ethics/ecode.htm

Americans with Disabilities Act (ADA) home page
    http://www.usdoj.gov/crt/ada/adahom1.htm

Facts about ADA
    http://www.eeoc.gov/types/ada.html

Health Insurance Portability and Accountability Act
http://www.hhs.gov/ocr/hipaa

Law all Nurses Should Know
http://www.continuingeducation.com/nursing/lawstoknow/
elements.html

National Council of State Boards of Nursing
http://www.ncsbn.org

Nurses Service Organization: Avoiding breaches in confidentiality
http://www.nso.com/newsletters/features/breaches.php

Patient Abandonment State of New York FAQs
http://www.op.nysed.gov/nurseabandon-qa.htm

Patient Self-Determination Act
http://www.abanet.org/publiced/practical/patient_self_
determination_act.html

Patient's Bill of Rights
http://www.democrats.senate.gov/pbr
http://www.cancer.org/docroot/MIT/content/MIT_3_2_
Patients_Bill_Of_Rights.asp

Telemedicine Information Exchange
http://tie.telemed.org

Tort Reform: Evidence from States (pro & con)
http://www.cbo.gov/showdoc.cfm?index=5549&sequence=0

Joint Economic Committee (U.S. Congress)
http://www.house.gov/jec/tort.htm

CHAPTER

23

ETHICAL ISSUES IN NURSING LEADERSHIP

INTRODUCTION

Nurses constantly make ethical decisions, based on principles of right or wrong, when delivering patient care. Ethics is a complex area, and it becomes increasingly more complex as medical technology advances and requires difficult patient care decisions. This chapter provides definitions and outlines the foundational principles and actions that are part of a nurse leader's ethical decision-making process.

KEY POINTS

1. Definition of **ethics**. "the science that deals with the principles of right and wrong, good and bad, and governs our relationships with others and that is based on personal beliefs and values" (Sullivan & Decker, 2001, p. 71)

   A. **Bioethics**

      i. the ethics specific to health care

      ii. provide a framework for behavior in **ethical dilemmas** (when there is a conflict between two or more ethical principles)

B. The shadowland of ethical dilemmas

      i. in some health care situations, the distinctions between law and ethics may not be clear (for example, providing or withholding treatment of a terminally ill person)

      ii. in some cases, ethics and law may be congruent, while in other cases, ethics and laws are in conflict, for example, providing a blood transfusion to save the life of a critically ill child whose parents object to transfusion on religious grounds (Sullivan & Decker, 2001)

C. The American Nurses Association maintains a nine-point code of ethics (summarized below):

      i. nurses provide services with respect for human dignity and uniqueness of the individual

      ii. nurses are committed to the patient

      iii. nurses advocate for the patient

      iv. nurses assume responsibility and accountability for nursing judgments and actions

      v. nurses maintain competence in nursing skills and practice

      vi. nurses maintain positive environments for care

      vii. nurses participate in activities that contribute to ongoing development of profession

      viii. nurses participate in collaborative practice nurses are responsible for the profession

      ix. American Nurses Association, 2001

D. Traditional **ethical theories**

      i. utilitarianism

        a. decisions based on what will provide the greatest good for the greatest number of people

        b. for example, the decision to force people with pulmonary tuberculosis into treatment is ethical, according to this theory, because it protects the greater population from infection

      ii. teleology (or consequentialist theory)

        a. value of a situation is determined by its consequences

        b. thus the outcome, not the action itself, is what counts; sometimes referred to as the "all's well that ends well" ethical approach

      iii. deontology (or formalism)

        a. an act is good only if it springs from goodwill

        b. this ethical theory does not allow for actions based on the concept of "the end justifies the means" (Little, 2003)

E. Definition of morality

    i. **morality** is "behavior in accordance with custom or tradition and usually reflects personal or religious beliefs" (DeLaune & Ladner, 2002)

    ii. for example, in some cultures, a woman appearing in public without her head covered is immoral (and perhaps illegal), while in other countries, it is morally acceptable for a woman's head to be uncovered

F. The four characteristics of a person of **virtue** (possessing moral goodness, the quality of engaging in ethical thinking and actions)

    i. compassion: desire to alleviate suffering

    ii. discernment: possessing acuteness of judgment

    iii. trustworthiness: reliable and dependable

    iv. integrity: having and maintaining sound moral principles (Little, 2003)

G. Common ethical principles and rules (and nursing examples)

    i. **beneficence:** duty to do good to others; maintain a balance between benefits and harm
        a. provide all patients, including terminally ill, with caring attention
        b. treat every patient with respect and courtesy

    ii. **nonmaleficence:** principle of doing no harm
        a. observe safety rules and precautions
        b. keep skills up-to-date

    iii. **justice:** principle of fairness that an individual receives what is due, owed, or legitimately claimed
        a. treat all patients equally, regardless of economic or social background
        b. learn state and organization's laws for reporting abuse

    iv. **autonomy:** respect for individual liberty and person's right to self-determination
        a. ensure that patients have given informed consent to all procedures
        b. know laws governing advanced directives
        c. release patient information only with appropriate consent; protect patient privacy

    v. **fidelity:** the principle of keeping one's promise or word
        a. make sure all required contracts are completed
        b. follow through on actions promised

    vi. **respect** for others: right of people to make their own decisions
        a. provide people with information they need to make decisions

      b. avoid telling patients what they should do; instead, help them see available options and choices and make their own decision

  vii. **veracity:** obligation to tell the truth

      a. admit mistakes promptly

      b. refuse to participate in any type of fraud (Little, 2003)

2. Historical/philosophical influences guiding ethical perspectives and nursing practice

  A. Religious

     i. women (and some men) who became nurses in early days of the profession were often either vowed religious or trained in religious values

    ii. early nursing training emphasized on church-supported values of obedience, humility, and sacrifice

   iii. christian tradition enhanced opportunities for women to serve in this capacity (Donahue, 1985)

  B. Women's issues

     i. women have historically been the traditional caregivers to the helpless and sick, either within or outside the family

    ii. women have historically been perceived as more sensitive, nurturing, and caring (Little, 2003)

  C. Philosophy of nursing

     i. **philosophy is:** rational investigation of truths and principles of knowledge, reality, and human conduct

    ii. nurse's personal philosophy and experiences strongly affect nursing philosophy

   iii. nurse's personal philosophy needs to be compatible with that of the organization in which the nurse works (Little, 2003)

  D. Values

     i. **values** are personal beliefs about the truth of ideals, standards, principles, and behaviors that give meaning and direction to a person's life

    ii. **values clarification** is the process of analyzing one's values to better understand what is important

   iii. three steps to values clarification include

      a. choosing: assumes that choices are made freely and that in choosing, a person analyzes the consequences of other alternatives; for example, a nurse chooses not to take a procedural shortcut after thinking through the possible consequences, such as harm to the patient

    b. prizing: the beliefs that are selected are valued; for example, the nurse who does the procedure properly values "doing the job right" as well as values improved patient outcomes

    c. acting: the chosen beliefs are consistently demonstrated through a person's behavior; for example, the nurse consistently follows procedure and encourages others to do so as well (Raths, Harmin, & Simon, 1978, cited in Little, 2003)

E. Steps for ethical decision-making

    i. gather data and identify conflicting claims
    ii. identify participants
    iii. determine moral perspectives and development of participants
    iv. determine desired outcomes
    v. identify options
    vi. take action on the choice
    vii. evaluate outcomes of action chosen (Burkhardt & Nathaniel, 2002)

3. The role of the ethics committee in health care organizations

A. Special ethical issues encountered in health care settings

    i. cost containment vs. cost of available technology
    ii. questions that arise include
      a. When do we refrain from using technology?
      b. When do we stop using it once it is started?
      c. Who is entitled to the technology? Those who can pay? Those who are uninsured? Everyone, no matter what? (Schroeder, 1995)
    iii. patient rights: hospitals and care providers are legally and ethically obligated to uphold the following patient rights to:
      a. participate in treatment decisions
      b. provide informed consent to treatment
      c. receive considerate and respectful care
      d. review records
      e. be informed of hospital policies
      f. expect reasonable and appropriate continuity of care after hospitalization (American Hospital Association, 1992)

B. An ethical nurse leader is:

    i. responsible for creating an ethically principled environment
    ii. accountable for upholding standards of conduct set by the profession

    iii. persistent and committed to bringing about any change needed
    iv. dedicated to ethical principles
    v. responsible for determining the ethical behavior of those under the leader's supervision; this ethical behavior governs
        a. interactions with people requiring nursing care
        b. responsibility for maintaining competence in nursing practice
        c. responsibility for meeting health care needs of the public
        d. maintaining cooperative relationships with other nurses and other coworkers
        e. determining and implementing desirable standards of nursing practice and education (ICN Code for Nurses, 1973, cited in Little, 2003)

REVIEW ACTIVITIES

Questions

1. The science that deals with the principles of right and wrong is called:
    a. ethics
    b. philosophy
    c. psychology
    d. morality

2. In this ethical theory, decisions are based on what will provide the greatest good for the greatest number of people.
    a. nonmaleficence
    b. teleology
    c. formalism
    d. utilitarianism

3. A person who possesses moral goodness and engages in ethical thinking and actions is said to have:
    a. ethics
    b. virtue
    c. autonomy
    d. values

4. A person whose behavior is in accordance with custom or tradition is:
    a. moral
    b. ethical
    c. beneficent
    d. trustworthy

5. The ethical principle of doing no harm is called:
   a. beneficence
   b. nonmaleficence
   c. justice
   d. veracity

6. A nurse who keeps his word and follows through on promised actions is practicing which ethical principle?
   a. justice
   b. autonomy
   c. veracity
   d. fidelity

7. The process of analyzing one's standards and principles of behavior to better understand what is most important to that person is called:
   a. values clarification
   b. nursing philosophy
   c. ethical decision making
   d. personal morality

Critical Thinking Questions

1. You are in the ER when an 18-year-old man is brought in after being shot and having sustained a spinal cord injury. His breathing is becoming more labored and the team is deciding whether to perform endotracheal intubation to facilitate ventilation now, or to rush him to the OR where he can be intubated. The nurse tells his patient that he may need to have a tube in his windpipe to assist his breathing. The patient says, "If I am going to be paralyzed, I want to die. Don't do anything to save my life." Should the patient be intubated, or should the patient be allowed to die of respiratory failure? Describe the ethical dilemma faced here using the theories and principles discussed in this chapter.

2. Hospitals that perform organ transplants have special teams of health professionals that procure organs and actually do the transplant. Are these teams involved in the care of patients with severe head injuries that may be eligible to become organ donors with family consent? Why or why not?

3. An elderly retired couple is on vacation when they are in a crash in their car. The husband is critically ill and expected to die. The wife is in the orthopedic unit with multiple broken bones and in traction. Routine tests show that the husband has syphilis, for which the wife should be treated as a precaution. Should the wife be told that her dying husband has a sexually transmitted disease (her test was negative), or should she be given the antibiotic treatment without a specific explanation?

Discussion Questions

1. What difficult ethical dilemmas or decisions have you confronted in your life or work? How did you resolve them?
2. What are your most important personal values? How do they direct and/or give meaning to your life?
3. What are the values of your organization (school or organization in which you work)? Have they ever conflicted with your personal values?

Works Cited

American Hospital Association. (1992). *A patient's bill of rights* (revised). Chicago, IL: Author.

American Nurses Association. (2001). *Code of Ethics for Nurses with Interpretive Statements*. Silver Spring, MD: American Nurses Publishing Available at http://www.ana.org/ethics/chcode.htm

Burkhardt, M. A., & Nathaniel, A. K. (2002). *Ethics & issues in contemporary nursing* (2nd ed.). Clifton Park, NY: Thomson Delmar Learning.

DeLaune, S. C., & Ladner, P. K. (2002). *Fundamentals of nursing*. Clifton Park, NJ: Thomson Delmar Learning.

Donahue, M. P. (1985). *Nursing, the finest art* (2nd ed.). St. Louis, MO: Mosby.

International Council of Nurses (1973). *ICN Code for Nurses: Ethical concepts applied to nursing*. Geneva: ICN.

Little, C. (2003). Ethical dimensions of patient care. In P. Kelly-Heidenthal (Ed.), *Nursing leadership & management* (pp. 266–279). Clifton Park, NY: Thomson Delmar Learning.

Raths, L., Harmin, M., & Simon, S. (1978). *Values and teaching* (2nd ed.). Columbus, OH: Merrill.

Schroeder, S. A. (1995). Cost containment in U.S. healthcare. *Academic Medicine, 70*(10), 861–866.

Sullivan, E. J., & Decker, P. J. (2001). *Effective leadership and management in nursing* (5th ed.). Upper Saddle River, NJ: Prentice Hall.

Additional Resources

Fitzpatrick, J. (2004). Naming and taming our ethical dilemmas. *Nursing Education Perspectives, 25*(2), 57.

Fraser, K. D. (2004). Decision-making and nurse case management: A philosophical perspective. *Answers, 27*(1), 32–43.

Garrett, T. M., Baillie, H. W., & Garrett, R. M. (2001). *Health care ethics: Principles and problems* (4th ed.). Upper Saddle River, NJ: Prentice Hall.

Hartley, J. (2004). Analysis. DNR case highlights ethical dilemma. *Nursing Times, 100*(3), 10–11.

Kälvemark, S., Höglund, A. T., Hansson, M. G., Westerholm, P., & Arnetz, B. (2004). Living with conflicts-ethical dilemmas and moral distress in the health care system. *Social Science & Medicine, 58*(6), 1075–1085.

Killion, S. W., & Dempski, K. (2000). *Legal and ethical issues.* Thorofare, NJ: Slack, Inc.

Kuhse, H. (1997). *Caring: Nurses, women, and ethics.* Cambridge, MA: Blackwell.

Seedhouse, D. (2000). *Practical nursing philosophy: The universal ethical code.* Chicester, NY: John Wiley.

Spencer, E. M., et al. (2000). *Organization ethics in health care.* New York: Oxford University Press.

Web Sites

Patient Bill of Rights
http://www.ana.org/gova/federal/legis/106/pbrintr.htm

International Centre for Nursing Ethics
http://www.freedomtocare.org/iane.htm

Nursing Ethics
http://www.nursingethics.ca

Nursing Ethics at Boston College School of Nursing. *Nursing Ethics* (journal)
http://www.arnoldpublishers.com/journals/pages/nur_eth/09697330.htm

Nursing Philosophy
http://www.blackwellpublishing.com/journal.asp?ref=1466-7681

Virtual Mentor: Ethics Journal of the American Medical Association
http://www.ama-assn.org/ama/pub/category/3040.html

Part VI

Putting it All Together and Becoming a Nursing Leader

CHAPTER

24

TEN WAYS TO BECOME A LEADER

Ten ways to become a leader regardless of job title, role or external sources of power

1. Make a commitment to lifelong learning

In the mid 1970s when many of today's nursing leaders were beginning their practice, there were no CT scanners, smoking was allowed in hospitals, and patients stayed in the hospital for three to four weeks after heart bypass surgery. There was neither AIDS nor bioterrorism.

Nurses must make a commitment to lifelong learning. One of the most exciting things about nursing practice is being part of such a dynamic field. However, being part of the health care team means having the responsibility to keep up-to-date with new developments in both nursing and health care.

Subscribe to a general nursing journal and one in a specialty area of interest. Attend continuing education programs and take advantage of the wealth of online learning activities.

2. Learn to write well

On a daily basis, nurses communicate through the written word by documenting care. It is critically important that nurses know how to write well. Having writing skills will reduce the risk of misunderstandings when documenting patient care and in writing notes and e-mail to others.

The best way to learn to write is to take courses in writing and composition whenever possible, and to write every day. Keep a journal about your experiences as a nurse or student.

Learn how to write about patient care situations so that you can share your challenges with others who can learn from your experience. As long as there is no identifying information about a particular patient, you can and should share your patient case studies. Physicians do this all the time in professional journals to describe unusual situations and how others can use the case study to improve their own practice. Virtually all nursing journals publish well-written case studies, and it is an ideal way to begin a publishing career. Editors at the general nursing journals (*American Journal of Nursing, Nursing 2006,* and *RN*) will assist novice authors who have a good story to tell about a challenging patient, how the nursing care team met the challenge, and what they learned.

3. Join a professional nursing association

Professional organizations are ideal places to meet other nurses with similar interests and to meet nurses who have a special commitment to the profession. Joining a national organization will also provide the option to join a local affiliate, which maybe a state or local group.

If you are interested in a particular specialty practice, joining the specialty organization is a way to learn more about the area of practice, to receive the specialty journal, and to meet people in the field.

Many nursing leaders hone their skills and their sphere of influence by meeting and working with nurses outside their organization through membership in professional associations. Building a network of nurses in the area through the association also provides chances to learn about employment opportunities and may also be a way to find a professional mentor.

4. Get involved in the community

Nurses are consistently ranked as the most honest and ethical of the professions in the annual Gallup Poll. The community already respects nurses, and nurses can have a great impact by volunteering in the community. Nurses have a wealth of skills, and they are not just bedside caretakers. Nurses are well organized, they know how to direct teams, and they perform well under pressure, just to name a few.

There are a wide variety of activities that are a good match for nurses' skills. Working at a health fair sponsored by your employer, providing general health screenings at the homeless shelter, and teaching CPR for the American Red Cross are just samples of the many activities that await a nurse's contribution. Your imagination is the only limit to what you can accomplish and how you can make a difference in your community—either by yourself or by coordinating activities with nursing colleagues.

5. Teach

Nurses teach all the time whether they realize it or not. When they explain why they are giving a particular medicine to a patient, or showing a family member how to hold the hand of a comatose patient, or demonstrating how to use crutches, they are effective teachers.

Make a commitment to the profession by teaching. If you are uncomfortable standing up in front of a group, start by offering to be a preceptor or resource person for a new staff member. Reach out to students who are on the nursing unit, offer to answer questions, and help them feel a part of the team.

When you teach, you are planting seeds for the future of the profession. Start your garden today.

6. Get politically involved

People in elected office are responsible to their constituents. Nurses can have significant power in the political arena if they communicate with their elected officials and provide the unique insight nurses have in health care issues. Two important pieces of federal legislation that were passed in the Congress were spearheaded by nurses: needlestick protection and the Nurse Reinvestment Act that provides money for nursing education.

Local involvement is just as important—changes to the Nurse Practice Act are made by state legislatures who need to learn about nursing practice and why proposed changes are good or bad for nursing. Local, regional, and state officials have a large role in determining how health care is funded, who is eligible for benefits, and how they are provided.

Learn who your elected officials are and communicate with them. You can telephone their offices, send e-mail, or make an appointment for a face-to-face meeting. Few citizens communicate with officials, so your voice will be amplified when you take the small effort to tell officials what is important to you as a nurse and to encourage them to support those positions.

7. Get certified

No matter where you practice, you can be certified in that practice area. Consumers are aware that physicians can be board certified, but few are aware that nurses can be as well. The more the nurses who support the profession by becoming certified, the more resources can be devoted to informing the public.

Certification is a tangible example of a nurse's commitment to lifelong learning and to validating knowledge gained during practice that goes beyond that tested on the entry-level NCLEX examination. Board certification tells the world that you are a professional registered nurse.

8. Serve on committees in your organization

Every organization has committees on which nurses can serve. Savvy nurses who want to be leaders join committees. Being a member serves two purposes: nurses make contributions to the organization, and they get known within the organization. When opportunities are present in the organization, offers are more likely to be made to nurses who are visible and known for service beyond work on the unit.

Choose a committee that has members from different departments besides nursing to gain a broader perspective on the organization beyond the nursing department and to get to know leaders in other areas. It will allow you to coordinate multidisciplinary care more effectively in the future and will build bridges that can help solve problems on behalf of patients and make care more efficient.

9. Give yourself a break

Nursing is the toughest career you will ever love. But, there are limits in the human condition and nurses who ignore that simple fact are doomed to burnout. Being burned out is not just being tired, it is being completely drained of the capacity to care and to be objective about the patient challenges nurses face. That is a dangerous place for a nurse to be.

If the organization in which you work is consistently understaffed and you are continually stressed, it may be time to move on. Similarly, if you are working with a group of nurses who are not professionals and whose values are very different from yours, look for another job in which you can thrive and be the nurse you want and know who you can be.

Nurses need to get a break from patient care and from giving. Be selfish. Take time for yourself. Develop a couple of hobbies that have nothing to do with health care or service that give you joy. It maybe singing in a choir, gardening, crafts, or playing sports, or a hundred other things.

The most important aspect of nursing is not to confuse being a nurse with having to be a Superman at the same time.

10. Be proud to be a nurse

As nurses, we are privileged to be there when patients are completely unprotected, naked, and vulnerable. What happens during those times between the patients and their nurses? It is recalled in a silent, knowing glance, with the assurance that those secrets are forever held within the glass that encases the innermost fears and dreams and knowledge in a nurse's soul. Nurses are the custodians of life crisis; we are the foremost patients' advocates.

Nurses change people's lives every day. Patients are comforted when they recognize your voice and say, "That's my nurse." They trust you; they believe in you.

Being a nurse is a privilege. The faith our patients place in us is a solemn trust that few other people will ever know. Be proud of what you do, the people you touch, and the lives you save. That's the mark of a true leader.

ANSWER KEY

Chapter 1

1. c	3. d	5. b	7. b	9. c
2. b	4. d	6. a	8. d	10. b

Chapter 2

1. a	3. c	5. b	7. c	9. a
2. c	4. d	6. b	8. a	

Chapter 3

1. b	3. d	5. a	7. b
2. a	4. c	6. a	8. c

Chapter 4

1. b	4. d	7. c	10. c
2. c	5. d	8. a	11. c
3. c	6. b	9. c	12. a

Chapter 5

1. c	3. c	5. b	7. a
2. a	4. d	6. a	

Chapter 6

1. d	4. c	7. b	10. a
2. c	5. d	8. d	11. c
3. c	6. d	9. b	12. b

Chapter 7

1. a	3. b	5. d	7. c	9. d
2. b	4. a	6. b	8. a	

Chapter 8

1. b	3. d	5. c	7. b	9. b
2. c	4. d	6. a	8. c	

Chapter 9

1. a	3. c	5. d	7. c	9. d
2. b	4. a	6. c	8. a	

Chapter 10

1. b	3. c	5. a	7. a
2. c	4. d	6. a	

Chapter 11

1. c	3. a	5. a	7. b
2. b	4. b	6. d	8. c

Chapter 12

1. b	3. d	5. c	7. b
2. a	4. a	6. a	

Chapter 13

1. c	3. a	5. b
2. a	4. c	6. a

Chapter 14

1. b	3. c	5. c	7. b	9. c
2. c	4. a	6. d	8. a	

Chapter 15

1. a	3. b	5. a	7. a	9. c
2. d	4. d	6. b	8. b	10. d

Chapter 16

1. b	3. c	5. a	7. b
2. c	4. d	6. b	

Chapter 17

1. c	3. b	5. d	7. a	9. b
2. b	4. b	6. a	8. a	10. b

Chapter 18

1. d	2. c	3. a	4. c	5. b

Chapter 19

1. a	3. b	5. a	7. c
2. b	4. c	6. c	8. a

Chapter 20

1. d	3. c	5. d	7. b	9. a
2. d	4. b	6. c	8. b	

Chapter 21

1. c	2. a	3. d	4. a	5. b

Chapter 22

1. b	3. a	5. a	7. b	9. a
2. b	4. b	6. c	8. b	10. c

Chapter 23

1. a	3. b	5. b	7. a
2. d	4. a	6. d	

INDEX

Abstract
  random channel, 143. (*See also* Gregorc
    Style Delineator)
  sequential channel, 143. (*See also*
    Gregorc Style Delineator)
Acceptance, expressing, 84
Accommodating, 125, 128–29. (*See also*
    Conflict: resolution methods)
Accountability, 53–55
  and leadership, 55–56
  consumer demand for, 56
  other aspects of, 56–57
Accountability-based care, 150, 153
Accuracy, 62
Accurate words, 67–68
Acknowledgement of message and
    feelings, 83
ACLS. (*See* Advanced cardiac life support)
Action
  evaluate, 95
  implementation, 94
Active learner's preferred style, 190
Active listening, 80–81
  effective, principles for, 83
  encouraging, 134
Adjourning, 140. (*See also* Team: develop-
    ment process)
Administration, 210, 213–16. (*See also*
    Health: professional groups)
Administrative law, 277
Administrative theory, 18, 23
Adult
  learners, 186, 189–91
  learning, stages of, 189–90
Advanced
  cardiac life support, 204
  practice nurse, 267, 270
Advocacy, consumer-oriented, 233–34
Advocate, political, 233
After the fact analysis, 175

Agency for Healthcare Research and
  Quality, 167, 221
AHRQ. (*See* Agency for Healthcare
  Research and Quality)
Ambulatory care centers, 212–13
American Nurses Association, 165,
  201–202, 247
  Credentialing Center, 204
  ten-point code of ethics, 297
ANA. (*See* American Nurses Association)
Analyze, 92
Androgynous, 86
Anger, 80, 86. (*See also* Emotions)
Appreciation, expressing, 84
Approval seekers, 132–33. (*See also*
    Difficult people, dealing with)
Arbitration, 241, 244
Arbitrator, 241, 244
Assertiveness, 80, 84–85
Assessment, 116, 253–54. (*See also* Change:
    process steps)
Associations, professional nursing,
  202–203
Attending. (*See* Active listening)
Attorney, consulting and collaborating
  with an, 290
Audience link, 66. (*See also* Cognitive
    management apparatus)
Auditory communication channel, 62, 65
Authorities, opinions of, 166
Authority, 2–3
  power, 44
Autocratic leadership, 2, 6
Autonomy, 296, 298–99
Avoiding, 125, 128. (*See also* Conflict:
    resolution methods)

Balanced scorecard concept, 180
Bargaining agent. (*See* Unions)
Barriers, 80, 85–87

Behavior link, 66. (*See also* Cognitive management apparatus)
Behavioral theories. (*See* Leadership: theories)
Benchmarking, 163, 167, 179
Beneficence, 296, 298
Benefits, 92, 94. (*See also* Decision-making)
Bennis and Nanus, 41
Big picture perspective, 100–101
Bioethics, 296–97
Biological variations, 85. (*See also* Culture)
Blaming, 80, 86, 133. (*See also* Emotions; Conflict: resolution, rules for effective)
Body language, 62, 68–69
Books, 201–02. (*See also* Publishing)
Brainstorming, 99, 101–2
Bureaucratic theory, 18, 22–23

Capitation, 210, 217
Care
    evidence based, 221
    planning and documentation, 73. (*See also* Nursing: information systems)
Care delivery
    management tools for, 192–94
    models, 186, 193
Case management, 53–54, 155–56, 186, 192–93, 267
Case managers, nurses as, 269
Case method, 193
CCRN. (*See* Critical care nursing)
CEN. (*See* Certified: emergency nurse)
Center for Medicare and Medicaid Services, 156
Cerebral elements of the brain, 142. (*See also* Hermann Brain Dominance Model)
Certainty, 92, 95. (*See also* Decision-making)
Certification, 201, 204, 267–68
    advantages of, 268
    to contract, 243
    getting, 307
    organizations sponsoring, 268
Certified emergency nurse, 204
Certified nurse midwife, 271
Certified registered nurse anesthetist, 271
Chain of command, 53
    effective use of, 56–57
Change, 109
    agent, 109–11

characteristics and strategies, 112–13
communication plan for facilitating, 118–20
managing, 118–19
process steps, 116–18
project team, 119. (*See also* Change: managing)
reactions to, 116
reasons to introduce, 111
recognizing impact, 119
types of , 110
Channels, 62, 65
Chaos theory, 109, 115–16
Charge nurse, 30, 33–34
Charisma
    power of, 40, 42–44
    theory of, 2, 9
Charting, 279–80
    do's, 279
    don'ts, 279
    by exception, 276, 280
    omissions, common, 279–80
    rules, 279
Chief nurse executive, 30, 33
Chronic wound management, 169
Civil law, 276–77
Clarifying, 80–82
Clinical experience, 253
Clinical nurse specialist, 270–71
Clinical pathways, 186, 192
Clinical practice council, 154. (*See also* Professional: practice structure)
Clinical skills, 186–87
Clowns, 141. (*See also* Dysfunctional: team roles)
Coercive power, 40, 45–46
Cognitive management apparatus, 62, 66–67. (*See also* Targowski-Bowman model)
Collaborating, 125, 130. (*See also* Conflict: resolution methods)
Collective bargaining, 241–43
    disadvantages of, 245
    federal regulation of, 242–43
    future of, 248
    issues, 248
    pros and cons, 244–45
    units for nurses, 247–48
Committee, 138–39
    serving on organizational, 307
Communication, 62–73
    barriers, 80, 85–87
    diagonal, 62, 70

Communication (*continued*)
   direct, 62, 64
   downward, 62, 70
   effective nurse-physician-patient,
      280–81
   electronic, 72
   future trends affecting, 87–88
   horizontal. (*see* Lateral communication)
   lateral, 62, 70
   models, 62, 65–67
   modes, 67–69
   nonverbal, 62, 68–69
   with patients and families, 71
   paths within organization, 70–71
   process, 62–63
   public, 71
   settings, 69–71
   skills
      advanced, 84
      basic, 80–85
      using to help process change, 119–20
   tools, 72–73
   upward, 62, 70
   verbal, 62, 67–68
   writing direct, 64
   written, 72, 305–306
Community, 53, 55
   involvement in, 306
Competency, 150, 154
Competing, 125, 129. (*See also* Conflict:
      resolution methods)
Complainers, chronic, 132. (*See also*
      Difficult people, dealing with)
Compliant behavior category, 142
Compromising, 125, 129. (*See also* Con-
      flict: resolution methods)
Conceding, 80, 86. (*See also* Emotions)
Concrete random channel, 143. (*See also*
      Gregorc Style Delineator)
Concrete sequential channel, 143. (*See
      also* Gregorc Style Delineator)
Conflict, 80, 86, 125
   dealing with, 82–83, 119
   definition, 125–27
   managing, 86. (*See also* Gender)
   resolution methods, 125, 128–30
   rules for effective resolution, 133–34
   types of, 127–28
Confronting, 125, 130. (*See also* Conflict:
      resolution methods)
Confusion, acknowledging, 120. (*See also*
      Change: managing)
Connectedness, 31

Connection power, 40, 43, 45
Consensus, 92, 98
Consequences, 92, 94. (*See also* Decision-
      making)
Consistency, creating, 119. (*See also*
      Change: managing)
Constituents, 53–54
Consumer demand, 53, 56
Consumer groups, skills to establish
      partnerships with, 234–35
Consumer-oriented advocacy, 233–34
Contemporary theories, 9
Continence nurse specialist, 271
Contingency theories, 2, 7–9
Continuous Quality Improvement, 18, 21
Contract administration, 244
Controlling, 18, 20–21
Cooke et al., 169
Coordinating council, 154. (*See also* Pro-
      fessional: practice structure)
Coordinator, 140. (*See also* Functional
      team roles)
Corporate structure, changes affect on
      nursing environments, 111–12
Cost-driven changes, 219–20
Costello-Nickitas, 41
Cost-reduction strategies, 217
Covey, Stephen, 41
CQI. (*See* Continuous Quality
      Improvement)
Creator, 140. (*See also* Functional team
      roles)
Criminal law, 277
Critical care nursing, 204
Critical outcomes, 99
Critical thinking, 92–93
   effective, 93
Criticizers, 141. (*See also* Dysfunctional:
      team roles)
Cultural diversity, 87
Culture, 80, 85, 126. (*See also* Communi-
      cation: barriers; Conflict)
Curiosity, 2, 4
Customers, 174, 176

Daring. (*See* Curiosity)
Decision-making, 18, 21, 92–93
   and technology, 99
   characteristics of, 93
   differences between novices and
      experts, 96–97
   ethical, steps for, 300
   factors affecting, 21–22

within groups, 97–99
    leadership/management issues
        and, 97
    and patient care, 97
    skills, 93–99
    strategic steps, 94
    successful, characteristics of, 93
    support systems, 62, 73
Decision tree, 92, 97, 99
Delegatee, 253–54
    accountability, 260–61
    choosing the right, 260–61
    job role expectations, 261
    providing feedback to, 261–62
    roles, 260
Delegating leadership style, 7
Delegation, 20, 253–62
    in action, 260–62
    and the individual, 258
    benefits of, 258
    communication role and, 261
    cultural differences and, 261
    definition, 253
    effective, outcomes of, 255
    five rights of, 255
    legal issues and, 258–60
    obstacles to, 255
    process, evaluating the, 262
    reluctance to, 258
    successful, keys to, 253–55
Delineate, 80, 82
Delphi group, 92, 98
Democratic leadership, 2, 6
Demographics, 231–32, 267
    changes and trends, 256
Deposition, giving a, 286
Desire, 2, 5
Detailers, 141. (See also Dysfunctional:
        team roles)
Diagnosis-related groups, 210, 217–18
Diagonal communication, 62, 70
Differentiated practice method, 193
Difficult people, dealing with, 131–33
Direct communication, 62, 64
Directing, 18, 20
Disagreement, 125–26
DISC behavioral model, 142
Discharge planning, 73. (See also Nursing:
        information systems)
Disciplinary procedures, 276
    understanding, 285–86
Distractions, controlling or minimizing,
        104

Diversity, 87. (See also Communication:
        future trends affecting)
Do not resuscitate (DNR) orders, 276,
        288
Documentation, 276, 279
Dominant behavior category, 142
Dominators, 141. (See also Dysfunctional:
        team roles)
Downtime, using effectively, 103–4
Downward communication, 62, 70
DRGs. (See Diagnosis-related groups)
Dysfunctional
    conflict, 125–26
    team roles, 138, 141

Education
    continuing, 205
    council, 154. (See also Professional:
        practice structure)
Effective decision makers, 93, 96–97
Egotists, 131. (See also Difficult people,
        dealing with)
Electronic communication, 72
E-mail, 72
Emotional intelligence. (See People-based
        intelligence)
Emotions, 85–86
Empathy, 80, 83
Empirical-rational change strategy,
        109, 113
Employee-centered leadership, 2, 6
Empowerment, 2, 9, 40, 46–48, 231
Entrepreneur, 267, 269–70
    benefits and challenges of, 269
    characteristics of a successful
        nurse, 270
    opportunities, 270
Environmental control, 85. (See also
        Culture)
Environmental factors, 22
Environmental link, 66. (See also Cogni-
        tive management apparatus)
Equity theory, 10–11
Ethical dilemmas, 296–97
Ethical practice. (See Principle-centered
        power)
Ethics, 296
    committee, role of, 300–301
    theories of, 296–98
Evaluate, 253–55
Evaluation, 117. (See also Change process
        steps)
    types of, 262. (See also Delegation)

Evidence-based care, 163–64
importance of, 165
Evidence-based practice
competencies, 163–64
development, 164
models, 163, 168–69
Executive information systems, 62, 73
Expectancy theory, 10
Expert
power of, 44
speaker as, 201, 204–6
Expertise, 40–42
developing, 154–55
External interference, 62, 64
Extrovert category. (*See* Myers-Briggs
type indicator)

Face to face
direct communication, 64
meetings, targeted, 118
Facial expressions, 69. (*See also* Body
language)
Facilitator, leader as, 143–45
deals with diversity, 145
full group promoter, 144
qualities of an effective, 144
responsibilities of a, 144
Familial diversity, 87
Family leave, 285
Featherbedding, 241–42
Feedback, 62–64, 80, 83, 195, 253
encouraging frequent, 134
providing to delegates, 261–62
types, 262
Feeling category. (*See* Myers-Briggs type
indicator)
Fidelity, 296, 299
Fielder's theory, 7. (*See also* Contingency
theories)
Financial pressures on health care
organizations, 256
Firefighter image, 19
Flexibility, 2, 4–5
Flight nurse, 272
FOCUS methodology, 174
five steps, 178–79
Focusing, 84
Follow-up, 134
Format, choose appropriate, 118. (*See also*
Change, communication plan for
facilitating)
Forming, 139–40. (*See also* Team: develop-
ment process)

Framework, 210
for quality health care, 222
FTE. (*See* Full time equivalent)
Full time equivalent, 186, 191
Functional nursing method, 193
Functions/role link, 66–67. (*See also* Cog-
nitive management apparatus)

Gantt chart, 92, 97, 99
Gender, 80, 86
studies, characteristics noted from, 11
Generalists, 31
Gestures, 68–69. (*See also* Body language)
Globalization, 223
Goal, 92, 94–95. (*See also* Decision-making)
setting theory, 11
Goals, 150–51
Good Samaritan laws, 276, 289
Government, 53, 55
Grapevine, 119. (*See also* Change:
managing)
information, 71
Gregorc Style Delineator, 143
Grief, anticipate, 120. (*See also* Change:
managing)
Grievance process, 241, 244
Ground rules, setting, 133
Group, 138–39
behaviors of, 141
decision-making in, 97–99
effective dependencies, 98
methods of, 98
obstacles to, 99
role of members in, 140–41
power of, 40, 45
Group meetings, 138, 145–46
focus, 146
managing dynamics in, 145–46
mobilization of, 146
preparation for, 145
Groupthink, 98
Guiding vision. (*See* Vision)

Havelock's six-step model, 114–15. (*See
also* Linear change theories)
Hawthorne effect, 18, 23
Health care
categories, 211–12
environment trends, 210, 218–20
environment, 210–11
environment, delegation and the,
255–58
framework for quality, 222

and nursing roles trends, 231–34
organization accountability, 55
organizations in the United States,
    212–13
payment, 216–17
recent changes in, 223–24
reform increases need, 256
Health Insurance Portability and
    Accountability Act, 158
Health maintenance organization,
    210, 217
Health professional groups, 213–16
Hermann Brain Dominance Model, 142
Hersey and Blanchard's situational
    theory, 7–8
Herzberg's theory, 24
Historical development, 164. (*See also*
    Evidence-based: practice develop-
    ment)
HMOs. (*See* Managed health care organi-
    zations)
Home health care agencies, 213
Honesty. (*See* Principle-centered power)
Horizontal communication. (*See* Lateral
    communication)
Hospice and Palliative Nursing position
    paper, 169
Hospital information systems, 62, 73,
    150, 156–57
Hospitals, 212
House's path-goal theory, 8
Humor, appropriate, 84
Human relations theory, 18, 23

Identify, 80, 82
Implementation, 117. (*See also* Change
    process steps)
Improvement, Model for, 167–68
Inattention, 80, 87
Incident reports, 280
Incidents, 280
Individual power, 40, 45
Informatics, 201, 204
Information giver/seeker, 141. (*See also*
    Functional team roles)
Information, power of, 40, 43
Information systems, 73
Influence, 40–41
Injunction, 241–42
Institution structure, 21
Integrated delivery systems, 219–20
Integrated health care systems, 210,
    218–19

Integrity, 2, 4. (*See also* Principle-
    centered power)
Intelligence, 2, 5
Interaction, 62, 64
Interactive behavior category,
    142
Interdisciplinary, 138
    teams, 139
Interference, 62, 64
Intermediate outcomes, 99
Internal interference, 62, 64
Interpersonal conflict, 125, 127–28. (*See
    also* Conflict: types of)
Interpersonal skills, 186–87
Interpreters, professional, 71
Interrupting, 80, 86–87
Interruptions, dealing with, 101
Intervene, 253–54
Intrapersonal conflict, 125, 127. (*See also*
    Conflict: types of)
Introvert category. (*See* Myers-Briggs
    type indicator)
Intuitive category. (*See* Myers-Briggs type
    indicator)
Inventory, 73. (*See also* Nursing: informa-
    tion systems)

JCAHO. (*See* Joint Commission on
    Accreditation of Healthcare
    Organizations)
Job descriptions, 195
Job discrimination, 284–85
Job performance, 186–87
Job safety, 34
Joint Commission on Accreditation of
    Healthcare Organizations, 31, 156,
    168, 179–80, 221
Journals, 202. (*See also* Publishing)
Judging category. (*See* Myers-Briggs type
    indicator)
Justice, 296, 298

Kerr and Jermier's substitutes for leader-
    ship theory, 8–9
Key themes, identifying, 134
Kinesthetic communication channel,
    62, 65

Labor-management committees,
    forming, 248
Laissez-faire leadership, 2, 6
Lateral communication, 62, 70
Laws, 276

Leader, 2–3
  distinguishing characteristics, 34–35
  ten ways to become a, 305–308
  traits of a, 4–6
  types of, 9
Leader-member relations, 7
Leadership, 2–3, 30–31, 40–41
  formal, 2–3
  gender, 5–6
  informal, 2–3
  roles, 35
  shared, 53, 55–56
  skills, 151
    using outside the health care organi-
      zation, 205–6
  style categories, 7–8
  successful, characteristics of, 3
  theories, 2, 6
    organizational changes effects
      upon, 12
  types, 2–3
Learning organization theory, 109, 116
Legal issues, 253
  and delegation, 258–60
Legitimacy, 40, 42
  power, 44
Lewin's Force-Field Model, 113–14. (*See
    also* Linear change theories)
Licensure, 258–59
Lifelong learning, commitment to, 305
Limbic elements of the brain, 142. (*See
    also* Hermann Brain Dominance
    Model)
Linear change theories, 109, 113–15
Lippitt's Phases of Change, 114 (*See also*
    Linear change theories)
Long-term care facilities, 212

Magnet status, 174, 181
Malpractice, 210, 221–22, 276–78
  insurance, 290
Managed care, 276
  legal risks/issues of concern,
    287–89
Managed health care organizations,
    213, 217
Management, 18–19, 30–31. (*See also*
    Supervision)
  council, 154. (*See also* Professional:
    practice structure)
  functions, 19–21
  information systems, 150, 156–58
    advantages of using, 157–58

disadvantages of, 158
  types of, 156–57
  without leadership, 26
  roles, 35
    factors affecting, 21–22
  stress, 54
  theories, current, 22
  traditional organizational, 24
Manager distinguishing characteristics,
    34–35
Managerial surveillance, 18, 21
Managing by objectives, 18, 20
Marquis and Huston, 127
Maslow's hierarchy of needs, 24
Mass catastrophe, 223
Matrix, 92, 97
Maximax approach, 92, 96. (*See also*
    Uncertainty)
Maximin approach, 92, 96. (*See also*
    Uncertainty)
MBO. (*See* Managing by objectives)
MBTI. (*See* Myers-Briggs type
    indicator)
McCarthy's 4-MAT model, 190
McGregor's theory, 24
Medicaid, 210, 216–17, 224
Medicare, 210, 216–17, 224
Medicine, 210, 213–16. (*See also* Health:
    professional groups)
Meetings, keeping on track, 102
Mentor, 186, 189, 210, 225
  professional, 102
Message, 62–63
Mind mediation channels, 143. (*See also*
    Gregorc Style Delineator)
Minority populations, 231–32
Mintzberg's model, 30, 34
Mission statement, 150–51
Mobilizer, 140. (*See also* Functional team
    roles)
Model for Improvement, 167–68
Models for moving research into
    practice, 169
Morality, 296, 298
Motivation, 186
  factors, 188
Motivational theories, 2, 9–11, 18,
    23–24
Multidisciplinary practice models,
    166–68
Multihospital systems, 219
Multistate practice/compact, 276, 289
Myers-Briggs type indicator, 142–43

Narrow span of control, 18, 21
National Council for Quality
  Assurance, 156
National Labor Relations Board, 241,
  243, 247
Nay-sayers, 132, 141. (*See also* Difficult
  people, dealing with; Dysfunc-
  tional: team roles)
NCAP. (*See* Noncredentialed assistive
  personnel)
NCQA. (*See* National Council for Quality
  Assurance)
Negators, 132. (*See also* Difficult people,
  dealing with)
Negligence, 276–77
Negotiating, 125, 129–30. (*See also* Con-
  flict: resolution methods)
Neonatal resuscitation program, 204
Networking, 186, 189
Neuro-linguistic programming, 190–91
New leadership concept, 2
Newsletters, 202. (*See also* Publishing)
NHPPD. (*See* Nursing hours per patient
  day)
NLRB. (*See* National Labor Relations
  Board)
Nominal group, 92, 98
Noncredentialed assistive personnel, 253
  roles of, 259–60
Nonlinear change theories, 109, 113,
  115–16
Nonmaleficence, 296, 298
Nonunion organization, 253
  delegation and, 257
Nonurgent outcomes, 99
Nonverbal communication, 62, 68–69,
  80–81, 83
Normative-reeducative change strategy,
  109, 113
Norming, 140. (*See also* Team: development process)
NRP. (*See* Neonatal resuscitation
  program)
Nurse advocate, ways of acting as a,
  235–36
Nurse
  as case manager, 269
  assignment, refusing an, 284
  collective bargaining units for, 247–48
  director, 30, 32–33
  disagreeing with a physician, 284
  entrepreneur, 269–70
  as expert witness, 286

flight, 272
leader
  accountability, 54–55
  characteristics, 31
  ethical, 301
  ways of acting as a, 235–36
manager, 30, 32
  roles and functions of, 31–33
  evaluating staff performance roles
    and responsibilities, 195–96
  as political advocate/activist, 233
  politically savvy, benefits of a, 232
  pride, taking, 308
  rights and responsibilities of, 281–84
  as sales representative, 269
specialist
  continence, 271
  flight, 272
  ostomy, 271
  wound, 271
  transdisciplinary trend, 224–25
  traveling, 267–68
Nurse Practice Act, 31, 259, 276–77
Nurse practitioner, 271
Nurses4Dean, 233
Nursing, 210, 213–16. (*See also* Health:
  professional groups)
  associations, professional, 202–203
  environments, change in, 111–12
  hours per patient day, 186, 191–92
  information systems, 62, 73, 150, 157
    applications, 157
  license, 276
    protecting, 285–87
  outcomes, 192
  practice 163–65
  primary, 53–54
  research, 163, 165–66
  role, trends affecting, 224–25
  shortages and opportunities, 267–69
  state boards of, 259
  trends, 210, 220–22
Nursing's ongoing dilemma, 24–25

Objectives, 18–19, 150–51
One person with the answer model, 56
Online Journal of Issues in
  Nursing, 202
Online publishing, 202. (*See also*
  Publishing)
Organization objectives, 21–22
Organizations
  change in, 109–10

Organizations (*continued*)
 conflict in, 125, 128. (*See also* Conflict:
   types of)
 hierarchies in, 69–70
 mentor role of, 225
 power of, 40, 45
 professional, 53, 55, 203
 roles in, 69
 structure of, 174, 176
Organizing, 18, 20
Ostomy nurse specialist, 271
Ouchi's theory, 24
Outcome, 92, 94–95. (*See also* Goal)
 critical, 101
 determining measurable, 156
 intermediate, 101
 monitoring, 174, 176
 nonurgent, 101
 nursing, 192
 optimal, 101
 patient, 192
 research, 163–64
Outside the box thinking, 188
Ownership, 174, 176–77

Pace, 62, 68
Pain management, 168
PALS. (*See* Pediatric advanced life
   support)
Paper trail, reducing, 102
Pareto principle, 99–100
Participating leadership style, 7
Partnership, 186–87
Partnerships, 231, 234–35
Passion, 2, 4
Passives, 141. (*See also* Dysfunctional:
   team roles)
Patience, 83. (*See also* Active listening)
Patient, 53
 accountability-based care, 54
 advocacy, 231, 233
 care
   delivery, first-line, 153
   issues, 276, 278–79
   link between decision-making
     and, 97
   management, 150–51
   quality improvement for, 177–78
   redesign method, 193
   services, vice president of, 30, 33
 classification, 73. (*See also* Nursing:
   information systems)
 injuries caused by, 281

outcomes, 192, 221
 satisfaction data, 180–81
 Self-Determination Act, 276, 281
Patient-focused care, 53–54, 150, 155
 method, 193
PDCA (plan, do, check, act) cycle, 174, 178
PDSA (plan, do, study, act) cycle, 163,
   167–68
Pediatric advanced life support, 204
Peer-review organizations, 217
People, dealing with difficult, 131–33
People-based intelligence, 5
Perceiving category. (*See* Myers-Briggs
   type indicator)
Performance
 improvement, 174–75
 management, using feedback for, 195
 measurement, 73 (*See also* Nursing:
   information systems)
   supporting staff excellence through,
     186, 194
 rewarding, 196
Performing, 140. (*See also* Team: develop-
   ment process)
Personal focus, 187–88
Personal space, issues of, 69
Personality, 126. (*See also* Conflict)
Perspective, 92–93
PERT. (*See* Program Evaluation and
   Review Technique flowchart)
PEW Health Professions Commission,
   224, 256
Philosophy, 296
 communicating your, 101
 influences on nursing, 299–300
Physical link, 66. (*See also* Cognitive man-
   agement apparatus)
Physicians and unions, 247
Placating. (*See* Conceding)
Plan, 253–54
Planning, 18–19, 117. (*See also* Change:
   process steps)
Point of service organizations. (*See* Man-
   aged health care organizations)
Point-of-care systems, 73. (*See also* Nurs-
   ing: information systems)
Political activist, nurse as a, 233
Political arenas, 231–32
Political lobbies, 231–32
Politics, 40, 47–48, 231
 and economics of human services,
   231–34
 getting involved in, 307

Populations
  aging, 87, 223
  minority, 231–32
Position power, 7
Positive interaction, 2–3
Posture, 69. (*See also* Body language)
Power, 40
  definitions of, 40–41
  guidelines for using positively, 44–45
  plus vision, 45
  positive sources of, 42–45
Power over, 40–41
Power with, 40–41
Power-coercive change strategy, 109,
    112–13
PPS. (*See* Prospective payment system)
Practice models, multidisciplinary,
    166–68
Pragmatist learner's preferred style, 190
Pressure ulcer management, 168–69
Preventive care, focus on, 220
Primary health care, 210–11
Primary nursing, 53–54
  method, 193
Principle-centered power, 40, 43–44
Prioritize work, six steps to, 101–2
Probability, 92
Process
  of influence, 2–3
  theories, 9–11
Processes, 174, 177
Professional associations, nursing,
    202–203, 306
Professional change, 109–10
Professional nursing organizations, 201
Professional organizations, 53, 55
Professional practice structure, 151–54
Program evaluation, 166
Program Evaluation and Review Tech-
    nique flowchart, 92, 97
Project management software, 99
PROs. (*See* Peer-review organizations)
Prospective payment system, 210, 217–18
Public
  communication, 71
  law, 276–77
Publishing, 201–202
Punishment power, 40, 45–46

QI. (*See* Quality improvement)
Quality assurance, 174–76
Quality council, 154. (*See also* Profes-
    sional: practice structure)

Quality improvement, 73
  definition, 174–75. (See also Nursing:
      information systems)
  evolvement history, 175
  examining efforts, types of data
      used, 181
  general principles of, 176–77
  information, gathering and sharing,
      180–81
  priorities, 176
  strategies, 178–80
Quality-of-life issues, 54
Questioning, 80–81

Reassurance, 84
Receiver, 62–63
Reciprocal, 2–3
Recorder, 140. (*See also* Functional team
    roles)
Referent power, 40, 42–44
Reflective learner's preferred
    style, 190
Re-forming, 140. (*See also* Team: develop-
    ment process)
Refreezing, 114
Regulatory requirements, 174, 179
Reinforcement theory, 10
Relating to others, 86. (*See also* Gender)
Religious diversity, 87
Rephrasing, 80–81
Representation election, 241, 243
Research
  council, 154. (*See also* Professional:
      practice structure)
  moving into practice, 169
Resolve, 80, 82–83
Resource nurse. (*See* Charge nurse)
Resources, adequate, 118. (*See also*
    Change, communication plan for
    facilitating)
Respect, 296, 299
Responding, 80–81
Responsibility, 53–54
Restating, 81
Reward power, 40, 46
Risk, 92, 95. (*See also* Decision-making)
  adjustment, 210, 221
  averting approach, 92, 96. (*See also*
      Uncertainty)
  management, 276, 290
Rogers' Diffusion of Innovations, 115.
    (*See also* Linear change theories)
Roles, in team, 70–71

Sales representative, 267
  nurses as, 269
Scientific management, 18, 22
Secondary health care, 210, 212
Self-confidence, 2, 5
Self-education, 201 203–4
Self-reliance, 31
Self-respect, protecting, 133. (*See also*
      Conflict: resolution, rules for effec-
      tive, 133–34
Selling leadership style, 7
Sender, 62–64
Sensing category. (*See* Myers-Briggs type
      indicator)
Sentinel event, 174, 179–80
Session link, 66. (*See also* Cognitive man-
      agement apparatus)
Sexual harassment, 276, 284–85
Shared governance, 150–54
Shared leadership, 53, 55–56
Shift summaries, 103
Situational leadership, 150, 154–55
Skills, using opportunities to increase or
      practice, 104
Sneaks, 131–32. (*See also* Difficult people,
      dealing with)
Social organization, 85. (*See also* Culture)
Social structure factors, 22
Socialization, 18, 20–21
Solutions, developing alternative, 134
Space, 85. (*See also* Culture)
Speaking style, 86. (*See also* Gender)
Specialists, 31
Speed. (*See* Pace)
Spoken message content, 86. (*See also*
      Gender)
Stabilization, 117. (*See also* Change:
      process steps)
Staff
  excellence, strategies for developing,
      188–91
  nurse, 30, 34
  performance, 186–91
      definition, 186–87
      development levels, 187
      evaluating, 195–96
      leadership's role in, 187
Staffing, 18, 20, 186, 191
  effective, evaluating, 192
  needs, 191–92
Stakeholders, 92, 97
State nursing board decisions, 286
Steady behavior category, 142

Stereotyping, 80, 86
Storage/retrieval link, 66. (*See also* Cog-
      nitive management apparatus)
Storming, 140. (*See also* Team: develop-
      ment process)
Storyboard, using a, 180
Strategic choice model, 66
Strategic planning, 150–54
  components of, 151
Stress, 80, 86
  management of, 54
Strike, 241, 245
Studies
  individual experimental, 165. (*See also*
      Nursing: research)
  meta-analysis of multiple controlled,
      165. (*See also* Nursing: research)
  nonexperimental, 166. (*See also* Nurs-
      ing: research)
  Quasi-experimental, 166. (*See also*
      Nursing: research)
Subacute care facilities, 212
Subject-based intelligence, 5
Sullivan and Decker, 41, 44
  principles of effective communication,
      63–64
Supervision, 18–19, 253–54. (*See also*
      Management)
Supervisor, 241
  definition, 245–47
Support, 2, 5
SWOT analysis, 150–51
Symbols link, 66. (*See also* Cognitive
      management apparatus)
System, 174, 177
Systems link, 66. (*See also* Cognitive man-
      agement apparatus)

Targowski-Bowman model, 62, 66–67
      (*See also* Cognitive management
      apparatus)
Task force, 138–39
Task structure, 7
Tax Equity and Fiscal Responsibility
      (TEFRA) Act of 1982, 217–18
Teams, 138–41
  development process of, 138–40
  function of, 139–40
  nursing method, 193
Team-building tools, 138, 142–43
Teams, type of 139
Technical skills, 186–87
Telemedicine, 276, 288

Telephone
  Efficient communication by, 101
  triage by, 276, 280
Telling leadership style, 7
Temporary service agencies, 213
Tension-breaker, 141. (*See also* Functional
      team roles)
Tertiary health care, 210, 212
Theorist learner's preferred style, 190
Theory Z. (*See* Ouchi's Theory)
Thinking category. (*See* Myers-Briggs
      type indicator)
Three "Ps", 47
Time
  and motion studies, 18, 22
  creating, 103
  nursing use of, 100
Time management, 99–104
  skills, 99–100
  strategy, effective, 100
  workplace strategies, 102–3
Timeline, map out a, 118. (*See also*
      Change: managing)
Timing. (*See* Pace)
Tone, 62, 68
Tools, 62
  for staying focused, 102
Tort, 276–77
Total
  patient care method, 193
  quality management, 174–75
TQM. (*See* Total quality management)
Traditional organizational management,
      24
Training, 126. (*See also* Conflict)
Transactional leader, 9
Transdisciplinary nursing, 224–225
Transformational leadership theory, 2, 9
Traveling nurse, 267–68
Trends in health care and nursing roles,
      231–34

UAN. (*See* United American Nurses)
Uncertainty, 92, 95–96. (*See also* Decision-
      making)
Unfreezing, 113
Union busting, 243

Unionization
  and professionalism, 246–48
  nurse manager's role in, 246
  process of, 243
Unionized organization, 253
  delegation and, 257
Unions, 241–42
  physicians and, 247
Unit-based quality improvement, 156
United American Nurses, 247
University of Colorado hospital model,
      166–67
Upward communication, 62, 70

Values, 296
  clarification, 296
  link, 66. (*See also* Cognitive manage-
      ment apparatus)
Veracity, 296, 299
Vice president of patient care services,
      30, 33
Victims, 132. (*See also* Difficult people,
      dealing with)
Virtue, 296
  four characteristics of, 298
Vision, 2, 4, 40
  articulate, 118. (*See also* Change:
      managing)
  power plus, 45
  statement, 150–51
Visual communication channel,
      62, 65
Vocabulary, 62, 68
Voice mail, 72–73

Web-based information, 73
Wheatley's new leadership theory, 11
Whistleblowing, 241, 246
Wide span of control, 18, 21
Withdrawers, 133. (*See also* Difficult
      people, dealing with)
Word choice, 62, 67
Words, accurate, 67–68
Workplace advocacy, 241, 245–46
Wound nurse specialist, 271
Writing direct communication, 64
Written communication, 72